HEALTH TECH BOOK SERIES

THE 50 MIRACLE CURES OF CORIANDER

FAST SOLUTIONS FOR DIABETES, HIGH BLOOD PRESSURE, CHOLESTEROL, GOUT, SLIMMING, KIDNEY, LIVER, JOINTS, ULCER, COLON …

BY

Professor Awad Mansour

Professor of Chemical & Pharmaceutical Engineering
Formerly with
University of Akron
OH, U.S.A.

First Edition
2009

HEALTH TECH BOOK SERIES
9923 S. Ridgeland Ave. STE 209
Chicago Ridge, IL. 60415

HEALTH TECH BOOK SERIES

Published and Printed in the United States by:
Health Tech Book Series

Mansour, Awad
THE 50 MIRACLE CURES OF CORIANDER

First Edition
ISBN: 9-6539-4392-1
EAN: 978-1-4392-6539-0

HEALTH DISCLAIMER

THE 50 MIRACLE CURES OF CORIANDER: IS DESIGNED FOR INFORMATIVE PURPOSES ONLY AND ANY READER IS EXPECTED TO CONSULT HIS FAMILY DOCTOR BEFORE TAKING ANY CHEMICAL OR NATURAL PRODUCTS AND THE AUTHOR IS NOT RESPONSIBLE FOR THE USE OR MISUSE OF THE INFORMATION CONTAINED WITHIN.

Table of Content

ITRODUCTION 5

CORIANDER AND ACNE 7

CORIANDER AND ANEMIA 11

CORIANDER AND ARTHRITIS 15

CORIANDER AND BLADDER INFECTION...........................19

CORIANDER AND BODY ODOR & BAD BREATH 23

CORIANDER AND CANCER...25

CORIANDER AND CELLULITE 27

CORIANDER AND CHOLESTEROL 31

CORIANDER AND CONSTIPATION....................................35

CORIANDER AND DENGUE FEVER....................................39

CORIANDER AND DIABETES..41

CORIANDER AND DIGESTION..47

CORIANDER AND DYSENTRY 49

CORIANDER AND EYE WASH & CATARACT 51

CORIANDER AND FEVER 53

CORIANDER AND GOUT 55

Coriander and Hair Loss Remedy With Coconut Oil and Lime...................59

CORIANDER AND HEART HEALTH 61

CORIANDER AND HEMORROHIDS 65

CORIANDER AND HYPERTENSION...................................69

CORIANDER AND INSOMNIA...73

CORIANDER AND IRRITABLE COLON 75

CORIANDER AND JAUNDICE 77

CORIANDER AND KIDNEY HEALTH 79

CORIANDER AND LIVER CIRRHOSIS 83

CORIANDER AND LOST APPETITE 89

CORIANDER AND MEMORY 91

CORIANDER AND MENSTRUAL FLOW PROBLEMS 93

CORIANDER AND MOUTH ULCER 95

CORIANDER AND NOSE BLEED...99

CORIANDER AND ODEMA (SWELLING) 101

CORIANDER AND PIMPLES, BLACKHEADS AND DRY SKIN 105

CORIANDER AND PROSTATE HEALTH 107

CORIANDER AND PROSTATITIS...111

CORIANDER AND PSORIASIS 115

CORIANDER AND SEX...119

CORIANDER AND SMALLPOX 123

CORIANDER AND SORE THROAT 125

CORIANDER AND TRIGLYCERIDES 127

CORIANDER AND ULCER 131

CORIANDER AND URINARY TRACT INFECTION (UTI) 135

CORIANDER AND WEIGHT LOSS 139

CORIANDER AS AN EFFICIENT HEAVY METALS DETOX SORBENT........143

CORIANDER CABBAGE MIRACLE SLIMMING SOUP 145

CORIANDER, LICE AND DANDRUFF 147

CORIANDER, NAUSEA AND VOMITING 149

CORIANDER PERFUMES AND COLOGNES...153

Coriander & Coca Cola Secret Formula 155

Phytochemical Compounds Inside Coriander & Their Effects on Health 157

Table of Content

ITRODUCTION 5

CORIANDER AND ACNE 7

CORIANDER AND ANEMIA 11

CORIANDER AND ARTHRITIS 15

CORIANDER AND BLADDER INFECTION 19

CORIANDER AND BODY ODOR & BAD BREATH 23

CORIANDER AND CANCER 25

CORIANDER AND CELLULITE 27

CORIANDER AND CHOLESTEROL 31

CORIANDER AND CONSTIPATION 35

CORIANDER AND DENGUE FEVER 39

CORIANDER AND DIABETES 41

CORIANDER AND DIGESTION 47

CORIANDER AND DYSENTRY 49

CORIANDER AND EYE WASH & CATARACT 51

CORIANDER AND FEVER 53

CORIANDER AND GOUT 55

Coriander and Hair Loss Remedy With Coconut Oil and Lime.................59

CORIANDER AND HEART HEALTH 61

CORIANDER AND HEMORROHIDS 65

CORIANDER AND HYPERTENSION 69

CORIANDER AND INSOMNIA 73

CORIANDER AND IRRITABLE COLON 75

CORIANDER AND JAUNDICE 77

CORIANDER AND KIDNEY HEALTH 79

CORIANDER AND LIVER CIRRHOSIS 83

CORIANDER AND LOST APPETITE 89

CORIANDER AND MEMORY 91

CORIANDER AND MENSTRUAL FLOW PROBLEMS 93

CORIANDER AND MOUTH ULCER 95

CORIANDER AND NOSE BLEED...99

CORIANDER AND ODEMA (SWELLING)..101

CORIANDER AND PIMPLES, BLACKHEADS AND DRY SKIN 105

CORIANDER AND PROSTATE HEALTH 107

CORIANDER AND PROSTATITIS...111

CORIANDER AND PSORIASIS 115

CORIANDER AND SEX...119

CORIANDER AND SMALLPOX 123

CORIANDER AND SORE THROAT 125

CORIANDER AND TRIGLYCERIDES 127

CORIANDER AND ULCER 131

CORIANDER AND URINARY TRACT INFECTION (UTI) 135

CORIANDER AND WEIGHT LOSS 139

CORIANDER AS AN EFFICIENT HEAVY METALS DETOX SORBENT........143

CORIANDER CABBAGE MIRACLE SLIMMING SOUP 145

CORIANDER, LICE AND DANDRUFF 147

CORIANDER, NAUSEA AND VOMITING 149

CORIANDER PERFUMES AND COLOGNES......................................153

Coriander & Coca Cola Secret Formula 155

Phytochemical Compounds Inside Coriander & Their Effects on Health 157

INTRODUCTION
Why I Wrote This Book?

The major reason behind writing this book about CORIANDER is the continuous success stories I received from my patients about the miracle results of using coriander for numerous health conditions; one of these unique stories is the one found by my favorite patient Mrs. Aisha Khulaifi from Qatar who suddenly suffered from foot swelling and could not wear her shoes!!!!Mrs. Aisha is a highly educated pleasant woman who believes in natural alternative solutions for all human health problems and she together with her big family got beautiful results after they used our natural formulas for different disorders!!!! She called me when I was on my way from Amman to Dubai asking about fast solution for her foot. I asked her to use coriander seed tea 2 to 3 times daily for 3 days.

She called me the second day full of joy and said" **Aim flying in the sky!!!!!**" My foot problem has been solved fast and I am able to wear my shoes easily in less than 24 hours!!!!!!

A second story was told to me by a lady from Emirates; she was suffering from back and joint pains and called me asking about solution. I asked her to take coriander tea for 4 weeks. She called me after 3 weeks only!!!She was shocked by the results; **all pains disappeared from the whole body** and she got other beautiful findings; **she lost some of her extra weight!!!!!**

Many other stories about using coriander seed tea as a diuretic and carminative tool for hypertension (high blood pressure) and for renal (kidney) failure!!!! Many hypertensive cases used coriander seed tea from kitchen together with my powerful PRESS OIL which is used externally 5 times daily as a relaxing agent. All cases including myself got rid of high blood pressure for good in less than 24 weeks!!!! I discovered myself with high blood pressure of 190/105 and I started to take my relaxation oil (PRESS OIL) together with coriander tea and after 12 weeks only I measured my blood pressure and found it normal!!!!!Now my pressure reads 120/80 and sometimes 110/70 without any medications!!!!!

Two Qatari patients with renal failure; one was on dialysis and the other was about to start dialysis: both avoided dialysis after starting taking coriander tea together with our food supplement RENO TECH and asparagus soup!!!

Huge number of people who got benefits of coriander for high lipid, cholesterol, diabetes, gout, colon disorders, joint pain, weight loss, skin disorders and many other health problems!!!!

I thank ALMIGHTY ALLAH for helping me learn the phytochemisty of herbs and computer to help people from many deadly health problems and I feel it is my responsibility to spread my experience among all people in the world.

Prof. Dr. Awad Mansour

Chicago, United States

November 2009

CORIANDER AND ACNE

Major Causes of Acne

Acne is known to be partly hereditary. Several factors are known to be linked to acne:

Family/ Genetic history, Hormonal activity, such as menstrual cycles and puberty. Inflammation, skin irritation or scratching of any sort will activate inflammation. Stress. "increased acne severity" is "significantly associated with increased stress levels, Hyperactive sebaceous glands, Bacteria in the pores, Use of anabolic steroids, Exposure to certain chemical compounds. Chloracne is particularly linked to toxic exposure to dioxins, namely Chlorinated dioxins, chronic use of amphetamines or other similar drugs.

Sulfur is probably the oldest acne remedy known to medicine and its origins as an anti-acne treatment.

Some famous products in the market use **Benzoyl Peroxide** or **Salicylic acid** but both chemicals cause many side effects and skin irritation!!!!

Coriander serves both as an herb and a spice. It is a healing herb that is used effectively in different parts of the globe. While Indians use it for its anti-inflammatory properties, many other nations use this perennial herb for acne.

A teaspoon of **coriander juice**, mixed with a pinch of **turmeric powder**, is another effective home remedy for acne pimples and blackheads. The mixture should be applied to the face after thoroughly washing it every night. **Mint juice** can be used in a similar manner as coriander juice.

Natural Methods of Treating Acne:

You can find full details of our natural protocol of treating acne problems in our book: **How to Rid Acne in One Week without Medications** which will be printed in the United States soon.

We can draw the main guidelines of our protocol as follows:

1. Juice that Heal: Coriander juice (mixed with turmeric powder or mint juice) is used as a treatment for acne, applied to the face in the manner of toner.

2. Food that Heal: Lettuce, Cucumber, Curcumin are also helpful. Apple Cider Vinegar, **Baking Powder is well known by their effects on improving** acne.

3. Herbs that Heal. Coriander, Aloe vera: Neem, Turmeric, Papaya., Calendula, Propolis is one of the best herbs for acne.

4. Milk that Heals: Camel milk (as narrated by Prophet Mohammad (PBUH) offers endless health benefits. One of those is treating acne. My patients who took 2 glasses of camel milk daily for 3 weeks found miracle results for acne!!!!!

5. Herbal Tea that Heals: Hundreds of acne cases who took our herbal tea composed of Lemon Balm and Coriander seed for 3 weeks could easily solve their acne without medications!!!!!

6. Food Supplemnts that Heal:, Vitamin B3, Zinc, MSM together with chlorophyll food supplement.

7. Essential Oils that Heal: Citronelol, a component of essential oils in **coriander**, is an excellent antiseptic. In addition, other components have anti microbial and healing effects which do not let acne go worse. Our oil: **Relax U:** was successfully used by acne patients!!!

8. Soap that Heals:Dr.Mansour Miracle Nano Soap was successfully used by hundreds who got rid of their acne in 7-10 days!!!!

9. Ceam that Heals: Many acne patients used our Cellu Tech cream which is used for fatty cellulite got rid of their acne in 3 weeks.

10. Bath that Heals: Many patients cured their acne by using a 15-minute baking powder bath together with our dead sea salt or mud!!!

CORIANDER AND ANEMIA

Anemia is a sign of few diseases and also diseases in itself. Anemia has been identified as a reduction of hemoglobin in the blood, which carries oxygen throughout the body. Anemia occurs when there is bleeding, when bone marrow cannot produce enough red blood cells, when those produced have a defect, or when something interferes with the survival of red blood cells. Iron-deficiency anemia, caused by heavy or recurring bleeding, is the most prevalent form of the disorder. Persistent bleeding may occur from the digestive tract and is associated with diseases like gastritis, ulcerative colitis, hemorrhoids, hematuria (urine bleeding), inflammatory bowel disease, including leukemia and kidney disease, can produce anemia. Some types of anemia can be traced to genetic disorders. In children and adolescents, anemia can often be traced to insufficient dietary intake of iron. Loss of blood in menstruation is typically the cause of anemia among girls and women. In men, chronic occult bleeding in the gastrointestinal tract often leads to iron deficiency anemia. Signs and symptoms of anemia include fatigue, pallor, irritability, loss of appetite, backaches, headaches, soreness in the mouth and breathlessness. The homeopathic science suggests that deficiency should have to be corrected by necessary dietetic supplements.

Eating foods that contain adequate, easily absorbed sources of iron may be the best policy for anemia prevention. A balance diet that provides the Recommended Daily Allowance of iron is generally sufficient to guard against anemia. Certain chemicals interfere with iron absorption, for example, tannin in tea, polyphenols in coffee, and cadmium in cigarettes. Avoid these items those interfere iron absorption. Other important nutrients are **folic acid**, used by bone marrow to produce blood, and **vitamin B12**. Your diet should contain the following beverages in order to prevent Anemia:

Coriander is good in iron content which directly helps curing anemia.

The iron content in coriander could prevent blood loss from excess bleeding.

From the phytochemical composition of coriander we can notice a number of chemical compounds forming Coriander act as excellent source of iron, which clearly means that coriander is a good candidate to be safely used for anemia!!!.

Coriander serves both as an herb and a spice. It is a healing herb that is used effectively in different parts of the globe. While Indians use it for its anti-inflammatory properties, many other nations use this herb for anemia.

We have many successful stories about using **coriander seed tea for anemia!!**

Natural Methods of Treating Anemia:

You can find full details of our natural protocol of treating anemia problems in our book:

How to Fix Your Anemia in One Week without Medications which will be printed in the United States soon.

We can draw the main guidelines of our protocol as follows:

1. Juice that Heal: Wheatgrass, Grape, Beet and Black Currant juice can be very helpful.

2. Food that Heal: *Sweet Potato, Beet, and Tomato are also helpful.* **Black Seed and Fenugreek** *are useful to solve anemia problem by the scientific research.*

3. Herbs that Heal: *Eating 1 tsp of alfalfa seed fenugreek and black seed every morning for 3 months is good for anemia.*

4. Milk that Heals: *Camel milk (as narrated by Prophet Mohammad (PBUH) offers endless health benefits. One of those is treating anemia problems. My patients who took 2 glasses of camel milk daily with black seed **for** 3 months found miracle results for both anemia and sex!!!!!*

5. Herbal Tea that Heals: *Hundreds of anemia cases who took our herbal tea ;**Circu Tech Tea** which is simply composed of Nettle, Wormwood, Black Currant, Alfalfa and **Coriander seed** for 3-6 months could easily solve their anemia problem without medications!!!!!*

6. Food Supplemnts that Heal: *Many patients obtained excellent results by using our food supplement named: **Circu Tech** which contains a number of **iron-rich** herbs including **Coriander seed!!**Together with **chlorophyll, folic acid and Vitamin B12 food** supplements.*

CORIANDER AND ARTHRITIS

Arthritis is inflammation of one or more joints, which results in pain, swelling, stiffness, and limited movement. There are over 100 different types of arthritis.

Symptoms

If you have arthritis, you may experience:

Joint pain, Joint swelling, Reduced ability to move the joint, Redness of the skin around a joint, Stiffness, especially in the morning, Warmth around a joint

From the phytochemical composition of coriander we can notice a number of chemical compounds forming Coriander act as excellent anti-arthritic agent, which clearly means that coriander is a good candidate to be safely used for arthritis, rheumatism, joint and back pain!!!.

Coriander serves both as an herb and a spice. It is a healing herb that is used effectively in different parts of the globe. Indians use it and its oil for its anti-inflammatory properties, arthritis back pain, joints pain and gout.

The therapeutic properties of Coriander essential oil are as an **analgesic**, aphrodisiac, antispasmodic, carminative, depurative, deodorant, digestive, carminative, fungicidal, lipolytic, revitalizing, stimulant and stomachic. Coriander oil can be useful to refresh and awake the mind. It can help for mental fatigue, migraine pain, tension and nervous weakness. **Coriander oil's** warming effect is also helpful for alleviating pain such as **rheumatism, arthritis and muscle spasms**.

There are some indications that are also can be useful in combating colds and flu.

Many stories successfully used coriander seed tea as an anti-arthritis together with our food supplement **Rheuma Tech** without any medications!!!!! One story was told to me by a lady from Emirates; she was suffering from back and joint pains and called me asking about solution. I asked her to take coriander tea for 4 weeks. She called me after 3 weeks only!!!She was shocked by the results; **all pains disappeared from the whole body** and she got other beautiful findings; **she lost some of her extra weight!!!!!**

Natural Methods of Treating Heart Problems

You can find full details of our natural protocol of treating arthritis problems in our book:

How to Rid Arthritis without Medications which will be printed in the United States soon.

We can draw the main guidelines of our protocol as follows:

1. Juice that Heal: Cranberry and **Celery juice** can be very helpful.

2. Food that Heal: Cherry, Lettuce, Cucumber, Cabbage and Tomato are also helpful. **Pomegranate, Ginger, Almonds** and **Walnuts** and **Grape Seed Extract, Baking Powder is well known by their effects on reducing arthritis and joint 3. Herbs that Heal:** Eating 1 tsp of alfalfa seed, Curcumin and ginger with honey every morning for 3 months is good for arthritis. The Indian herb; Shilajit is one of the best herbs for arthritis.

4. Milk that Heals: Camel milk (as narrated by Prophet Mohammad (PBUH) offers endless health benefits. One of those is treating arthritis problems. My patients who took 2 glasses of camel milk daily or our food supplement **Rheuma Tech** for 3 months found miracle results for both arthritis and sex!!!!!

5. Herbal Tea that Heals: Hundreds of arthritis cases who took our herbal tea ;**Uri Tech Tea** which is simply composed of Celery, Alfalfa, Parsley and **Coriander seed** for 3-6 months could easily solve their arthritis problem without medications!!!!!

6. Food Supplemnts that Heal: Many patients obtained excellent results by using our food supplement named: **Rheuma Tech** which contains a number of **anti-arthritic** herbs including **Coriander seed!!!!**

7. Essential Oils that Heal: A number of patients informed me about excellent results on their arthritic joints, back and knees by using my oil mix of coriander oil and mustard oil for 6 weeks only!!!Coriander oil stimulates circulation. Eases muscular stiffness. Relieves arthritis and inflammatory conditions.

CORIANDER AND BLADDER INFECTION

Bladder Infection (BI) is an infection by the bacteria of the urinary tract which includes kidney, ureters, bladder or urethra. The infection of the bladder can develop into cystitis-a very common problem faced by women. Bladder Infection can infect anyone but women are more susceptible to this disease. Children too suffer from this disorder but the headcount is very low in comparison to adults. Sexual intercourse is another reason for Bladder Infection.

From the phytochemical composition of coriander we can notice a number of chemical compounds forming coriander act as excellent diuretic anti-inflammatory agents, which clearly means that coriander is a good candidate to be safely used for Bladder Infection!!!.

Coriander serves both as an herb and a spice. It is a healing herb that is used effectively in different parts of the globe. While Indians use it for its anti-inflammatory properties, and hence for Bladder Infection.

Many stories about using coriander seed tea as a diuretic **and** anti-inflammatory tool for Bladder Infection!!!! Many Qatari and Saudi BI patients; got rid of it within 4 weeks only!!!!After starting taking coriander tea together with our food supplement **URI TECH** and **Cranberry Juice** without any medications!!!

Natural Methods of Treating Bladder Infection Problems:

You can find full details of our natural protocol of treating Bladder Infection problems in our book:

How to Rid Bladder Infection in 3 Weeks without Medications which will be printed in the United States soon.

We can draw the main guidelines of our protocol as follows:

1. Juice that Heals: Cranberry and drinking 2-3 glasses water on empty stomach can be very helpful.

2. Food that Heals: Lettuce, Cucumber, Cabbage are also helpful. Pomegranate, **Baking Powder is well known by their effects on improving** Bladder Infection.

3. Herbs that Heal: Eating 1 tsp of corn silk and cinnamon with honey every morning for 3 weeks is good for Bladder Infection. The Indian herb; Shilajit is one of the best herbs for BI. Dandelion and Tribulus **terrestris are also useful.**

4. Milk that Heals: Camel milk (as narrated by Prophet Mohammad (PBUH) offers endless health benefits. One of those is treating BI problems. My patients who took 2 glasses of camel milk daily or our food supplement **Uri Tech** for 3 months found miracle results for both BI and sex!!!!!

5. Herbal Tea that Heals: Hundreds of gout cases who took our herbal tea; Uri **Tech Tea** which is simply composed of Corn Silk, Parsley and Coriander seed for 3-6 weeks could easily solve their Bladder Infection problem without medications!!!

6. Food Supplemnts that Heal: Many patients obtained excellent results by using our food supplement named: **Uri Tech** which contains a number of diuretic herbs including Coriander seed!!!! together with **chlorophyll** supplement.

7. Essential Oils that Heal: You can make an essential oil by using equal parts of Coriander, sandalwood, frankincense and juniper. Mix all these ingredients to make an oil to be rubbed over your bladder area. Continue this massaging technique for three to four days once the symptoms subside

8. Avoid irritant foods: A diet which consists of processed food like cheese, chocolate, dairy products should be avoided. You should also avoid spicy food, caffeine, alcohol and cigarettes which otherwise is also harmful. Avoid carbonated drinks like beer, soda or any other drink with fizz, and Aspartame which is one of the artificial sweeteners.

CORIANDER AND BODY ODOR & BAD BREATH

Body odor can be unpleasant as well as embarrassing, and for some people, it is a constant worry. The smell of waste products excreted by our bodies is also affected by toxins we have ingested or absorbed into our bodies. In a modern environment, our bodies are subjected to a host of **chemicals and toxins** in our food - including pollution in the air and even household cleaning products. Alcohol and tobacco is known to contribute to bad body odor – so try to cut back or avoid smoking and drinking completely.

Coriander is also widely used to cure halitosis and bad breath in general.

Coriander Oil is a good deodorant too. It clears bad breath and eliminates mouth and body odor, when used internally or externally. When consumed or ingested, the typical aroma of this Coriander Oil mixes with the sweat and fights body odor as well as fights oral odor as its scent, coming up from your stomach, fills your mouth. This also helps inhibit the bacterial growth in mouth and around sweat glands and thereby fighting odor. Mixed in water, when externally applied or used as a mouthwash, it again does it all!!!

Coriander Oil cleans blood of toxins and thus acts as a detoxifier or blood purifies. It helps remove the regular toxins like uric acid, heavy metals and certain compounds and hormones produced by the body itself, from blood, as well as other foreign toxins which get into blood accidentally.

There are a number of other home remedies to rid bad odors from mouth and body such as:

Chlorophyll: To prevent body odor, drink a glass of water in the morning, on an empty stomach, along with 500 mg wheat grass. The chlorophyll present in the grass will help in reducing body and mouth odor.

Mint

Parsley

Green and Black Tea

Milk Thistle is very famous to remove toxins from the liver.

Zinc is also very beneficial for curing bad breath.

There are many herbs also which helps to remove the bad odor like rosemary, parsley. Spearmint and tarragon, these herbs help to freshen up your mouth.

Also make a solution of baking soda by adding water and do regular gargles from this solution. It can also clean the tongue. This is one of the excellent home based remedy to reduce the bad breath. You can also apply baking soda to your armpits as well as to your feet, to reduce body odor.

While bathing, add white vinegar or apple cider vinegar to a mug of water and use it to rinse the armpits. This will definitely help in lessening the body odor.

Mix 10 drops of the essential oil such as **Coriander oil**, Lavender or Bergamot oil in 30 ml water. Apply this mixture on the armpits to reduce body odor.

CORIANDER AND CANCER

Coriander is indigenous to southern Europe, but it is used widely in Asiatic and South American cuisine as well as that of the Mediterranean region. Coriander leaves are used to garnish salads and the roots feature regularly in Thai cooking. However, the small fruits (often called seeds) are the most important part of the plant and are a crucial ingredient of curry powders. Coriander is also used in a range of savory dishes, desserts and confectioneries, as well as in liqueurs and perfumes. The same is true from a medicinal perspective, as the fruits contain the highest concentrations of all the important phytochemicals that occur in this plant. While there is still limited understanding of the mechanisms through which coriander acts, initial research indicates that it is effective as both a treatment and preventive agent for several chronic diseases.

Cancer

Coriander's anti-tumorigenic properties have been demonstrated in relation to colon cancer. It works by protecting against the damaging effects of lipid oxidation associated with this malignancy. It is highly probable that coriander also contributes to the low incidences of several other cancer types seen in the populations of Eastern nations that consume large quantities of this spice.

Coriander Helps Fight Breast and Liver Cancers

Coriander is rich in coriandrol, which is believed to help combat breast and liver cancers. In animal studies, coriandrol stops aflatoxin from binding to DNA and causing liver cancer in some people.

CORIANDER AND CELLULITE

Mix base oil with **coriander**, thyme, and wintergreen or carrot essential oil and use to massage the cellulite affected area.

Diane Irons, author of Teen Beauty Secrets suggests rubbing warm coffee grounds into the fatty area.

Diane Irons also suggests rubbing down the body with Epson salts while in the shower to help with the cellulite.

It is suggested to use our cellulite oil and cream: **CELLU TECH** OIL AND CREAM which includes Coriander oil with strong massage to get excellent results.

From: sparkpeople.com: Lose inches & cellulite DIY Body Wrap and more Body wrapping is a therapeutic treatment that is used to detoxify the body using simple all natural ingredients. These simple readily available ingredients have been used over the years traditionally to tighten and tone the skin and help stimulate the body to rid itself of trapped toxins, excess fat and excessive trapped lymph fluids. This detoxification improves the appearance of cellulite, creates inch loss, and helps tighten and tone the skin.

HERBAL BODY WRAP RECIPE

Mix a cup of 369 corn oil with 1/2 cup of grapefruit juice and 2 teaspoons dried thyme. Massage into hip, thigh, and buttock areas. Cover with plastic wrap to lock in body heat.

(For extra results lay a heating pad over each area for five minutes)

CLAY BODY WRAP RECIPE

1 cup bentonite or green clay

1/4 cup sea salt

2 tbsp. olive oil

2 cups water

Boil water and add sea salt until it is dissolved. Add remaining ingredients and stir. Adjust the water if necessary to form a wet paste. Rub the mixture over your entire body and cover yourself with thin towels or a clean white sheet. Most salons will recommend that you use proper wrapping sheets as the compaction helps to squeeze the tissues together for greater results.

Lay in the tub for a minimum of 45 min. to one hour. Cellulite and Fat Fighting Ingredient Tips Coffee Grounds Rub coffee grounds on cellulite/fat area before taking a shower every night. The coffee helps firm the area and lessen that "cheese" look.

WHY?

Caffeine is the first ingredient in most cellulite treatments. The same way caffeine gets us moving in the morning, it can also help to get our fat cells moving. This trick, employed by famous models and beauty contestants, involves rubbing warm coffee grounds into the cellulite-laden areas of your legs, using your hands or a loofah mitt. To intensify the treatment, take a rolling pin and roll the area to further smooth out the cellulite.

Another Anti-Cellulite treatment with Caffeine

Put magazines or newspaper on the floor of your bathroom or if you would like not to mess again, get in the tub and get messy! Mix a 1/4-cup of warm used coffee grounds with one tablespoon of olive oil. Stand on the paper or sit in the tub and apply the coffee mixture to your cellulite areas using your hands or a loofah mitt. Don't worry if a lot of the coffee mixture falls to the floor or tub; don't worry if many coffee grounds fall as most will stick to your skin to do the trick.

Wrap the area in plastic wrap and allow to remain for several minutes (for as long as you can handle it). Remove wrap and shower with warm water. This procedure is most effective when repeated twice a week.

Drink Green Tea Daily: WHY?

According to research published in the American Journal of Clinical Nutrition "consumption of green tea produces thermogenesis and increases energy expenditure and fat oxidation in humans.

Green tea is an active ingredient used in many of the top weight loss products. When a weight loss product claims it contains natural ingredients, green tea is nearly always in the list. Did you know that?

Essential Oils for fighting Cellulite and Fat

Buy essential oils (they are cheap on EBay) and use them for a massage every day. If you hate the feel of oil, try adding the oils in a cream which you use as your moisturizer. A simple way to do this is to buy a fragrance-free lotion or cream (available at health food stores) and add 20 drops of essential oils per ounce of the product.

WHY?

The "bumps" of cellulite are composed of fat, cellular wastes and water. The oils used to counteract the condition improve circulation, strengthen connective tissues, encourage the elimination of wastes and fight fluid retention.

Experiment with the following oils: (Always use a carrier oil)

Defeat your cellulite and fatty areas with:

Basil, birch, cedar wood, clary sage, coriander, cypress, fennel, geranium, ginger, grapefruit, juniper, lemon, orange, patchouli, pine, rosemary, and thyme.

Always keep in mind, the essential oils need to be mixed ALWAYS with a carrier oil*. It is very dangerous to use essential oils on their own on your skin without mixing them with carrier oil. Please use caution

Examples of carrier oils are sweet almond, apricot kernel, grape seed, avocado, peanut, olive, pecan, macadamia nut, sesame, evening primrose, walnut and wheat germ.

Special Cellulite Massaging Oil

5 drops fennel oil

4 drops rosemary oil

2 drops coriander oil

4 drops lavender oil

Add these oils in 20 ml of carrier oil. Massage into affected area daily.

Moisturizer Cellulite Rub

2 drops bay oil

2 drops lemon oil

4 drops lavender oil

Add these oils in 20 ml of sesame oil. Massage into affected area daily.

Cellulite Cream

Add Algae Powder to any of your favorite body lotion/ cream. This combination will help reduce cellulite and water retention and it also aids in the reduction of toxins and stress.

Adding 2 tablespoons of this powder to your bath will leave both your body and mind free of impurities.

Cellulite Oils/Herbs: White Birch, Cypress, Sweet Fennel, Geranium, Grapefruit, Juniper, Lemon, Parsley, Rosemary, Thyme, Coriander.

CORIANDER AND CHOLESTEROL

Cholesterol is a fatty substance, also called a lipid, that's produced by the liver. It's also found in foods high in saturated fat, like fatty meats, egg yolks, shellfish, and whole-milk dairy products. It's a vital part of the structure and functioning of our cells. However, high levels of cholesterol in your blood may lead to the slow buildup of plaque in the arteries over time, a serious disease called atherosclerosis.

The fact is that cholesterol can be harmful to your health when there's too much cholesterol in your blood. Whether you have high cholesterol may depend on your lifestyle. Eating a lot of fats and not getting enough exercise can cause cholesterol levels to rise. Cholesterol is also, in part, a result of your genetic makeup.

Everyone with high cholesterol needs to keep it under control, but it may be even more important for some groups of people, such as

- People with a family history of early heart disease
- People with high blood pressure
- People with diabetes
- People with obesity
- People with continuous stress
- Males over age 45
- Females over age 55
- Smokers

From the phytochemical composition of coriander we can notice a number of chemical compounds forming Coriander act as anti-lipid and anti-cholesterol agents, which clearly means that coriander is a good candidate to be safely used for high cholesterol.

Coriander serves both as an herb and a spice. It is a healing herb that is used effectively in different parts of the globe. While Indians use it for its anti-inflammatory properties, many other nations use this perennial herb for high cholesterol.

In for high cholesterol management it has been shown that Coriander acts as an anti-lipid agent and also helps in the vasodilation of veins!!

Many high cholesterol cases used **Coriander seed tea** from kitchen together with my powerful **Choles Tech** food supplement and after 3 months they got excellent results without any medications!!!!!

Natural Methods of Treating High Cholesterol:

You can find full details of our natural protocol of treating high cholesterol in our book:

How to Lower Your High Cholesterol to Normal without Medications which will be printed in the United States soon.

We can draw the main guidelines of our protocol as follows:

1. Juice that Heal: Acai, Tomato, Cucumber, and Celery juice can be helpful.

2. Food that Heal: Dark Chocolate, Peanut Butter, Lettuce, Cucumber, Sunflower seeds, Yogurt and Tomato are also helpful. **Garlic** is useful to lower the blood high cholesterol by the scientific research. **Apple cider vinegar** to lower cholesterol: It is said that an 8oz.apple juice with a tablespoon of apple cider vinegar will lower cholesterol. Almonds and

Walnuts are very famous for lowering cholesterol._**Grape Seed Extract and Pomegranate are well known by their effect in lowering** cholesterol.

3. Herbs that Heal: Eating 1 tsp of flax seed and black seed every morning for 3 months is said to prevent high cholesterol due to heredity factors. They also cure high cholesterol due to obesity, as both seeds have weight reducing properties. The Indian famous herb; Guggul.

4. Milk that Heals: Camel milk (as narrated by Prophet Mohammad (PBUH) offers endless health benefits. One of those is treating high cholesterol. Camel milk is said to be the vasodilator of the Future". My patients who took 2 glasses of camel milk daily or our food supplement: **CholesTech** for 3 months found miracle results for both high cholesterol and sex!!!!!

5. Herbal Tea that Heals: Hundreds of high cholesterol cases who took our herbal tea ;**Heart & Love Tea** which is simply composed of Cinnamon, Fenugreek and **Coriander seed** for 3-6 months could easily reduce their high cholesterol to normal without medications!!!!!

6. Food Supplemnts that Heal: Many patients obtained excellent results by using our food supplement named: **Choles Tech** which contains a number of anti-lipid herbs including **Coriander seed!!!!**

7. Essential Oils that Heal: Our oil mix which includes Coriander Oil in it was successfully used with hundreds of high cholesterol patients together with Coriander tea and all of them became high cholesterol free!!!!!!

In a research paper authored by V. Chithra and S. Leelamma entitled "Hypolipidemic effect of coriander

seeds" The effect of the administration of coriander seeds (Coriandrum sativum) on the metabolism of lipids was studied in rats fed a high fat diet with added cholesterol. The spice had a significant hypolipidemic action. The levels of **total cholesterol and triglycerides decreased significantly** in the tissues of the animals of the experimental group which received coriander seeds.

A recent experiment from the Biochemistry Department at the University of Kerala, in India, studied the effects of coriander seeds on rats that had been fed a very high-fat, high-cholesterol diet. Researchers saw significant drops in total cholesterol and triglyceride levels in the rats as cholesterol was broken down faster and eliminated.

CORIANDER AND CONSTIPATION

Here are the best 12 herbal remedies for Constipation (see carihal.com):

12 Top and Best Constipation Cures:

Constipation refers to a health condition when fewer bowel movements are occurred than it should be. It is indeed an uncomfortable and embarrassing health situation that even require serious medical attention if continues for longer period. Typically, if you are having less than three bowel movements in a week, quite obviously you are suffering from constipation problem. However, lack of exercise and unhealthy diet can contribute to constipation development. Constipation is not a serious problem till it becomes chronic.

However not so serious at initial stages, but it is always better that you should find ways for constipation cure and apply them accordingly as required. This article focuses on various types of constipation cure and their associated benefits.

1.Triphala Since ancient times, Triphala is well respected for its various nutritional benefits including a sophisticated solution as constipation cure. Triphala is an Indian preparation that constitutes three herbal components, namely, Amalaki, Haritaki and Bibhitaki. Triphala serves the purpose of both purgative laxative as well as lubricating bulk laxative. So, if you are suffering from constipation problem, you can definitely count on Triphala as the best constipation cure. Triphala functions nicely even in the case of chronic constipation problem. It effectively cleanses the colon and digestive system. Hence it protects the body from harmful bodily wastages.

2. Psyllium husk This offers a special household solution to constipation cure. It is obtained from the seed of the Plantago ovata plant. In Ayurvedic literature, this herb has been illustrated as an emollient, fresh, gentle laxative and diuretic.

3.Bael Fruit Bael fruit is truly popular for its ability to combat constipation. If you are suffering from constipation problem and would like to count on Bael fruit while looking for a cure to constipation, you need to use this fruit in its raw form regularly, for at least 2 to 3 months of time, prior to either breakfast or meal.

4.Senna Identified in the name of Markandika in Ayurveda, Senna offers an ideal way to relieve constipation and encourage bowel movement smoothly.

5. Licorice: This is beneficial for softening the stools. Also it has nutritional value as it is rich in fiber content. It works very effectively if it is combined with Senna.

6. Coriander Leaves The primary function of this herb is to boost the digestive system.

7. Grapes Grapes are truly effective in treating constipation in addition to providing nutritional benefits. With its outstandingly delicious and sophisticated flavor, grapes offer an excellent solution for constipation treatment of both sorts, temporary and chronic.

8. Dandelion To drink a tea mixed with dandelion powder can restore your health. This is not amere saying, but in reality dandelion can offer you a miracle. It has the ability to promote bowel movement and offer you a relief from constipation problem.

9. Sweet Figs This is commonly used in the case of constipation. It has a traditional value. It is also effective in digestion problem.

10.Amaltas This is scientifically known as Cassia fistula. Its fruit is used, specifically the fruit pulp. You can mix the pulp with the lukewarm water and drink it on a regular basis. It will provide you a relief from constipation problem. It is also safe to use during pregnancy, however, seeking medical attention is always recommended.

11. Honey. Honey offers several health benefits and protects us from many health hazards. This is also true in the case of constipation. If you mix one teaspoon of honey in one cup of lukewarm water and drink it regularly in the morning before breakfast, you will certainly come out from your constipation problem.

12. PRUNE JUICE IS ONE OF THE BEST

CORIANDER AND DENGUE FEVER

Dengue is an acute infectious viral disease transmitted by the Aedes mosquitoes. Common in tropical climates, the dengue fever is also known as "break-bone fever" due to the severe joint and muscle pain suffered by the patients. Other symptoms of dengue include severe headache, fever, and intense joint pain, which will usually last about a week. The fever will usually subside after 2 to 5 days and thereafter will rise again followed by rashes on the skin. The dengue hemorrhagic fever is another form of the disease, which is more serious and can be fatal. More than 300, 000 patients in West Saudi are suffering from Dengue fever.

There is only one cure for Dengue fever which is MC10 herbal supplement which was very effective in curing all Saudi cases in 24 hours. The same product is used for Malaria.

There is a famous Coriander soup is extensively used for Dengue fever:

CRAB SOUP

First in my list would be the "Crab Soup", which is delicious and can be easily prepared. Believe me that after 3 servings of this crab soup, the patient's blood platelets will increase and fever will subside. Just give it a try.

Ingredients:

2 crabs which have been cleaned and cut into two (can be any type, for instance flower crab or tiger crab)

1 inch of ginger (cut into small pieces)

1 clove of garlic (crushed)

1 shallot (pounded)

Cooking oil (2 spoonful)

4 ounces of water

Salt

5 Peppercorns (pounded)

1 lemon grass (crushed)

Juice from 1 lime (squeezed)

1 strip each of **coriander** leaf and Chinese leak (cut into small pieces)

Directions:

Heat the cooking oil in a pot. Put in the shallot, garlic, ginger and peppercorn and fry (in low heat) until you can smell the sweet and tangy aroma.

Put in the crabs and flip the crabs occasionally until both sides turned red

Put in water and lemon grass

Turn the heat low and cover the pot with a lid. Bring the soup to boil for at least 15 minutes.

Put in the lime juice and some salt (as desired)

Stir the ingredients in the pot for 5 minutes

Put in the coriander leaf and Chinese leak on the dish

The soup is now ready to be served

CORIANDER AND DIABETES

From the previous chapter which discussed the phytochemical composition of coriander seed and leaf we noticed a number of compounds which are either anti-diabetic or hypoglycemic and in both cases coriander seed and leaf lower blood sugar if they are used as an herbal tea on daily basis. Moreover coriander contains anti-stress hypotensive vasodilating compounds which are responsible in enhancing blood circulation which in turn improves blood sugar levels and retards the diabetes consequences in eye vision, kidney and heart functions and improves sex and blood circulation to the foot and hence prevents diabetic foot gangrene.

Some other compounds of coriander raise the good cholesterol; HDL, and lowers bad cholesterol; LDL which may cause or worsen diabetes!!!!

Moreover some components of coriander like chromium are a famous mineral which improves insulin resistance for TYPE II diabetics!!!

Coriander serves both as an herb and a spice. It is a healing herb that is used effectively in different parts of the globe. While Indians use it for its anti-inflammatory properties, many European nations use this perennial herb for its anti-diabetic qualities.

In diabetes management it has been shown that Coriander acts in a manner similar to insulin and also helps in the secretion of Insulin (please see the paper authored by:Gray and Flatt from the University of Ulster, UK: Insulin-releasing and insulin-like activity of the traditional anti-diabetic coriandrum sativum (Coriander) published by Br.J.Nutrition; 81(3) (203-209)1999

Main types of diabetes:

Type 1 ("insulin-dependent" and previously called "juvenile diabetes"). Type 1 diabetes is associated with a partial or total damage of beta cells in the pancreas which do not produce enough amounts of insulin. It develops most often in children and young adults. Type 1 diabetes represents 5%-10% of diabetics and is traditionally treated with insulin.

Type 2 ("insulin-independent" or sometimes called "adult-onset diabetes"). Type 2 diabetes is associated with insulin resistant cells. It is much more common and usually develops in older adults. Type 2 diabetes represents 90-95% of diabetics.

Gestational (pregnancy-related). Some women develop diabetes during pregnancy. It affects 3 to 5 percent of all pregnant women. Although it goes away after pregnancy, these women have a higher chance for developing type 2 diabetes later in their lives.

Symptoms of Diabetes

Millions of people have diabetes and do not even know it because the symptoms develop so gradually, people often do not recognize them. Some people, particularly pre-diabetics, have no symptoms at all. Diabetics may have SOME or NONE of the following symptoms:

- Frequent urination
- Excessive thirst
- Extreme hunger

- Unexplained weight loss
- Sudden vision changes
- Numbness in hands or feet
- Poor blood circulation
- Poor sleep
- Feeling fatigue and tired most of the time
- Dry skin
- Sores that is slow to heal
- More infections than usual

Natural Methods of Treating Diabetes:

You can find full details of our natural protocol of treating diabetes in our book:

How to Lower Your Sugar from 400 to 100 without Medications which will be printed in the United States soon.

We can draw the main guidelines of our protocol as follows:

1. Juice that Heal: Wheatgrass, Tomato, Cucumber, Okra, celery and **Cabbage** juice can be helpful.

2. Food that Heal: Watermelon, Lettuce, Cucumber, Yogurt and Tomato are also helpful... Garlic and Onion are useful to lower the blood sugar by the scientific research. Apple Cider Vinegar on green salad is daily recommended

3. Herbs that Heal: Eating 1 tsp of curry leaves every morning for 3 months is said to prevent diabetes due to heredity factors. It also cures diabetes due to obesity, as the leaves have weight reducing properties. As the weight drops, the diabetic patients stop passing sugar in urine. Turmeric is one of the best spices that helps detoxify liver and lowers blood sugar!!!

4. Milk that Heals: Camel milk (as narrated by Prophet Mohammad (PBUH) offers endless health benefits. One of those is treating diabetes. Camel milk is said to be the Insulin of the Future". My patients who took 2 glasses of camel milk daily or our food supplement: **Camel Tech** for 3 months found miracle results for both diabetes and sex!!!!!

5. Herbal Tea that Heals: Hundreds of diabetics who took our herbal tea ;**Dia Tea** which is simply composed of Fenugreek, Cinnamon and **Coriander seed** for 3-6 months could easily reduce their blood sugar from 400 to 100 without medications!!!!!

6. Food Supplemnts that Heal: Many patients obtained excellent results by using our food supplement named: **GlucoLife** which contains a number of hypoglycemic herbs including **Coriander seed!!!!**

7. Essential Oils that Heal:

Coriander oil for type II diabetes

Name: Gloria Baswick

Location: Didsbury, Alberta, Canada

My mom was diagnosed with type 2 diabetes about 3 years ago. I immediately tried oils for her. First we tried dill -- no luck. Then we tried fennel -- it, too did not work. I then got some **coriander** for her and this has been amazing for her. She puts a drop on the inside of each ankle at bedtime and her blood sugars are always normal. She doesn't even watch her diet very closely (although the Dr. keeps saying 'You must really watch your diet -- your blood sugar is perfect!'

Researchers from the University of Cairo used **Coriander Oil** together with other essential oils and experimented them on diabetic mice and they got excellent results!!!!!

A Delicious Coriander Soup is recommended for Diabetics:

Asparagus with Mushrooms and Fresh Coriander Recipe

Ingredients:

1 lb Fresh Asparagus
2 tbsp Butter OR=
2 tbsp Margarine
1/2 lb Mushrooms, sliced (2 cups)
2 tbsp Shallots
1/2 tsp Salt
1 Freshly ground black pepper
4 tbsp Fresh coriander, chopped

Preparation:

Trim off tough part of asparagus stalk, about 2 to 3 inches from bottom. Use a vegetable peeler to scrap asparagus to about 1 inch from top. Cut asparagus on diagonal into 1 inch pieces. Melt butter in a non stick frying pan. Add mushrooms and cook over high heat, tossing and shaking, until mushrooms are lightly browned. Add asparagus. Cook, stirring and tossing for about 1 minute. Add shallots, salt and pepper. Sprinkle with coriander. Cook for 30 second and   serve.
Taking care of you naturally, the way life was meant by GOD!!!!

CORIANDER AND DIGESTION

Coriander, due to its rich aroma because of its essential oils, apart from being an excellent appetizer, helps in proper secretion of enzymes and digestive juices in the stomach, stimulates digestion and peristaltic motion. It is helpful in treating problems like anorexia.

Coriander's main reputation lies with its ability to support the digestive system. It is a fine stomach tonic that stimulates the secretion of gastric juices thereby helping to promote good digestion. Coriander is said to soothe the stomach of both adults and colicky babies and generally reduce irritation in the gastrointestinal tract, including heartburn(acid reflux), nausea and stomach pain.

Coriander serves both as an herb and a spice. It is a healing herb that is used effectively in different parts of the globe. While Indians use it for its anti-inflammatory properties, many other nations use this herb for digestion.

We have many successful stories about using **coriander** seed tea for digestion**!!**

Natural Methods of Treating Digestion:

You can find full details of our natural protocol of treating digestion problems in our book:

How to Fix Your Indigestion in One Week without Medications which will be printed in the United States soon.

We can draw the main guidelines of our protocol as follows:

1. Juice that Heal: Wheatgrass, Mint-Lemon juice can be very helpful.

2. Food that Heal: Okra is also helpful. Propolis and Licorice are useful to solve digestion problems by the scientific research.

3. Herbs that Heal: Eating 1 tsp of Lemon Balm, Mint, Ginger every morning for 3 months is good for digestion.

4. Milk that Heals: Camel milk (as narrated by Prophet Mohammad (PBUH) offers endless health benefits. One of those is treating digestion problems. My patients who took 2 glasses of camel milk daily for 3 months found miracle results for both digestion and sex!!!!!

5. Herbal Tea that Heals: Hundreds of anemia cases who took our herbal tea; Diges **Tech Tea** which is simply composed of Mint, Chamomile, Ginger, Lemon Balm and **Coriander seed** for 3 months could easily solve their digestion problem without medications!!!!!

CORIANDER AND DYSENTRY

Dysentery is not a disease but a symptom of a potentially deadly illness. The term refers to any case of infectious bloody diarrhea, a scourge that kills as many as 700, 000 people worldwide every year. Most of the victims live in developing areas with poor sanitation, but sporadic cases can pop up anywhere in the world.

People afflicted with amebic dysentery often suffer profuse, bloody diarrhea along with a fever, intense stomach pain, and rapid weight loss. Bacillary dysentery causes small, frequent stools mixed with blood and mucus. Cramps are common, and a patient may occasionally strain painfully, without success, to evacuate the bowels.

Coriander is a valuable herb in treating digestive disorders. One or two teaspoons of coriander juice, added to fresh buttermilk, is highly beneficial in treating indigestion, nausea, **dysentery**, hepatitis and ulcerative colitis. It is also helpful in typhoid fever. Dry coriander helpful to treat diarrhea and chronic dysentery, acidity. A Chutney made from dry coriander, green chilies, grated coconut, ginger and black grapes, without seed are a wonderful remedy for abdominal pain due to indigestion.

One teaspoon of **coriander powder** and sugar candy 3 times a day is an effective remedy to cure dysentery.

Home remedy for Dysentery:

50 gm Yogurt mixed with small amount of honey 3 times a day gives fast relief. Herbal decoction is prepared with two

tablespoons of dried out **coriander seeds**, and taken with pure water or buttermilk, the intestinal inside layer is soothed, and the amount of mucus in the stools declines. The use of pomegranate rind is an added effectual preparation for dysentery. About 60 grams of the rind should be boiled in the 250ml of milk. Apple is also considered advantageous in the management of acute and chronic dysentery in the kids.

Make a paste of curry leaves and black cumin seeds; consume this paste with a glass of boiled water.

Have sweet lemonade several times a day.

The following herbs, supplements, and dietary recommendations may also be a part of your treatment plan:

Garlic, Goldenseal, Black Walnut, Wormwood, Pumpkin Seed, Grape Fruit Seed.

Other natural remedies: Anise, Cloves, Gentian, Neem, Olive leaf, Oregano, Propolis, Thyme, Barberry, Oregon grape

CORIANDER AND EYE WASH & CATARACT

Conjunctivitis refers to an inflammation of the conjunctiva, the thin transparent membrane covering the front of the eye. This is also referred to as having 'sore eyes' and is a very common form of eye trouble. It spreads from person to person through direct Contact. Overcrowding, dirty surroundings and unhealthy living conditions can cause epidemics of this ailment. Conjunctivitis results from bacterial or a virus infection or eyestrain. Prolonged work under artificial light and excessive use of the eyes in one way or the other, no doubt, contribute towards the disease.

The eyeball and underside of the eyelids become inflamed. At first, the eyes are red and itchy. Later, there may be a watery secretion.

A decoction prepared from freshly dried **coriander** is an excellent eye-wash in conjunctivitis. It relieves burning and reduces pain and swelling

For Cataract: Mix 50 Gums of Anise**, Coriander** and Jaggery each. Take 12 Gms of this mixture thrice daily for three months. The symptoms of Cataract are resolved in 3 months.

1. Juice that Heal: Raw juices of certain vegetables, especially carrots and spinach, have been found valuable in conjunctivitis. The combined juices of these two vegetables have proved very effective. The juice of the Indian gooseberry, mixed with honey, is useful in conjunctivitis.

2. Food that Heal: Propolis is useful to solve conjunctivitis problems by the scientific research.

3. Herbs that Heal: Eyebright, Lemon Balm, Chamomile, Wormwood.

4. Herbal Tea that Heals: Coriander seed tea is recommended.

5. Vitamins that Heal: Vitamins A and B2 have proved useful in conjunctivitis.

6. Bath that washes and Heals: Chamomile extract is a fast healing bath on eyes lids.

CORIANDER AND FEVER

Ginger coffee: It is a Mixture of dried ginger and coriander seeds to be used as a coffee to promote health without side effects and reactions. Very good for digestion, cold, cough and fever.

Coriander seeds reduce fever and promote a feeling of coolness.

It also eases allergies and hay fever.

In any type of fever, Coriander adds to relief by inducing urination in a natural way. An Indian boiled mixture prepared out of Coriander, buttermilk, curry leaves, cumin seeds and is included in diet of a patient who is suffering from fever helps in reducing fever and supplying readily available calories to patient who is anorexic due to pyrexia.

If we take coriander tea prepared with coriander decoction, very little milk and sugar. This causes sweating and brings down temperature.

During summer, soak anise seeds, coriander seeds and poppy seeds overnight. In the morning, grind the seeds in the same water and filter it to obtain a super coolant drink for the body.

Natural Methods of Treating High Fever:

You can find full details of our natural protocol of treating high fever in our book:

How to Fix High Fever in 5 Minutes without Medications which will be printed in the United States soon.

We can draw the main guidelines of our protocol as follows:

1. Juice that Heal: Lemon-Mint juice can be very helpful.

2. Foods that Heal: Radish

3.Herbs that Heal: Aloe Vera, Chamomile, Gotu Kola, Lavender and Fenugreek

4. Herbal Tea that Heals: Hundreds of high fever cases who took our herbal tea ;**Fevo Tech Tea** which is simply composed of Violet, Chamomile and **Coriander seed** for 3 days could easily solve their high fever problem without medications!!

CORIANDER AND GOUT

Gout results from consuming rich foods loaded with urine that leads to an excess of uric acid, which can build up in the joints and crystallize, causing attacks of painful gout. The needle-like crystals inflame the body joints and cause severe stiffness, swelling and pain, particularly in the big toe, ankles, and feet. In the past, treatment of gout included severe dietary restrictions. Today, natural foods together with herbs can solve the gout problem.

Gout is known as the **"Disease of Kings"** because it is associated with persons of wealth, rich foods, red meat and excessive alcoholic consumption; gout (a form of arthritis) is identified with a number of well-known names in history. From among these are: King Henry VIII, Nostradamus, Isaac Newton, and Charles V, who ruled one of the largest empires in the world.

In controlling gout, high-protein foods increase the blood level of uric acid, and should be almost totally eliminated from the diet. Avoid purine-rich vegetables such as asparagus, cauliflower, dried beans, lentils, and peas; red meat.

As for drinks, one should avoid alcoholic drinks completely during a gout attack. However, one should drink plenty of fluids.

From the phytochemical composition of coriander we can notice a number of chemical compounds forming Coriander act as excellent **diuretic** anti-edema agents, which clearly means that coriander is a good candidate to be safely used for gout!!!.

Coriander serves both as an herb and a spice. It is a healing herb that is used effectively in different parts of the globe. While Indians use it for its anti-inflammatory properties, many other nations use this perennial herb for gout.

Many stories about using coriander seed tea as a diuretic and carminative tool for high uric acid**!!!!** Many Qatari and Saudi gout patients; got rid of it within 4 weeks only!!!! After starting taking **coriander tea** together with our food supplement **URI TECH** without any medications!!!!!

Natural Methods of Treating Gout Problems:

You can find full details of our natural protocol of treating gout problems in our book:

How to Get Gout out without Medications which will be printed in the United States soon.

We can draw the main guidelines of our protocol as follows:

1. Juice that Heal: Cranberry and **Celery juice** can be very helpful.

2. Food that Heal: Cherry, Lettuce, Cucumber, Cabbage and Tomato are also helpful. **Garlic** is useful to lower uric acid by the scientific research. **Pomegranate, Ginger, Almonds** and **Walnuts** and **Grape Seed Extract, Baking Powder is well known by their effects on improving kidney functions.**

3. Herbs that Heal: Eating 1 tsp of alfalfa seed and black seed every morning for 3 months is good for gout. The Indian herb; Shilajit is one of the best herbs for gout. **Dandelion and Tribulus terrestris are also very useful.**

4. Milk that Heals: Camel milk (as narrated by Prophet Mohammad (PBUH) offers endless health benefits. One of those is treating gout problems. My patients who took 2 glasses of camel milk daily or our food supplement **Uri Tech** for 3 months found miracle results for both gout and sex!!!!!

5. Herbal Tea that Heals: Hundreds of gout cases who took our herbal tea ;**Uri Tech Tea** which is simply composed of Celery, Alfalfa, Parsley and **Coriander seed** for 3-6 months could easily solve their gout problem without medications!!!!!

6. Food Supplemnts that Heal: Many patients obtained excellent results by using our food supplement named: **Uri Tech** which contains a number of **diuretic** herbs including **Coriander seed!!!!**Together with **chlorophyll** supplement.

7. Essential Oils that Heal: A number of patients informed me about excellent results on their gouty toes and knees by using my oil mix of coriander oil and mustard oil for 3 weeks only!!!1

Coriander and Hair Loss Remedy With Coconut Oil and Lime

Although hair is not essential to life, it is of sufficient cosmetic concern to provoke anxiety in anyone when it starts thinning, falling, or disappearing. To a woman, the sight of a comb or brush covered with lost hair can cause intense mental strain.

Hair is formed in minute pockets in the skin called follicles. An up growth at the base of the follicle, called the papilla, actually produces hair when a special group of cells turn amino acids into keratin, a type of protein of which hair is made. The rate of production of these protein 'building blocks' determines hair growth. The average growth rate is about 1.2 cm per month, growing fastest on women between fifteen to thirty years of age.

The most important cause of loss of hair is inadequate nutrition. Even a partial lack of almost any nutrient may cause hair to fall. Persons lacking in vitamin B6 lose their hair and those deficient in folic acid often become completely bald. But the hair grows normally after the liberal intake of these vitamins. Other important causes of loss of hair are stress such as worry, anxiety, and sudden shock; general debility caused by severe or long standing illnesses like typhoid, syphilis,, chronic cold, influenza, and anemia; an unclean condition of the scalp which weakens the hair roots by blocking the pores with the collected dirt; and heredity.

Directions for Use: Daily application of refined coconut oil, mixed with lime water and lime juice, on the hair, prevents loss of hair and lengthens it. Application of the juice of green coriander leaves on the head is also considered beneficial.

Expected Results Within: 1 month

(From: mamaherb.com)

CORIANDER AND HEART HEALTH

Everyone with heart problems needs to keep it under control, but it may be even more important for some groups of people, such as

- People with a family history of early heart disease
- People with high blood pressure
- People with diabetes
- People with obesity
- People with continuous stress
- Males over age 45
- Females over age 55
- Smokers

From the phytochemical composition of coriander we can notice a number of chemical compounds forming Coriander act as anti-lipid and anti-cholesterol agents, which clearly means that coriander is a good candidate to be safely used for heart disorders.

Coriander serves both as an herb and a spice. It is a healing herb that is used effectively in different parts of the globe. While Indians use it for its anti-inflammatory properties, many other nations use this perennial herb for heart health.

Heart Palpitation treatment using Aniseed and Dry Coriander

Palpitation of the heart may occur due to a variety of factors, most of which may not be related to the heart itself. Anything which increases the work load of the heart may bring on this condition. Some persons may experience palpitations when lying on the left side, because the heart is nearer the chest wall in that position. Many nervous persons suffer from this condition.

A mixture of powdered aniseed, dry coriander, and jaggery can also be used beneficially in the treatment of this condition. Equal quantities of each of these three substances should be powdered. About six grams of this mixed powder should be taken after each meal by the patient suffering from palpitation of the heart!!!!!!!

Palpitation is also treated by using Grapes, Honey, or Guava.

In for high cholesterol management it has been shown that Coriander acts as an anti-lipid agent and also helps in the vasodilation of veins!!

Many heart cases used **Coriander seed tea** from kitchen together with my powerful **Heart Life** food supplement and after 3 months they got excellent results without any medications!!!!!

Natural Methods of Treating Heart Problems:

You can find full details of our natural protocol of treating heart problems in our book:

How to Fix Your Heart without Medications which will be printed in the United States soon.

We can draw the main guidelines of our protocol as follows:

1. Juice that Heal: Noni, Tomato, Cucumber, and Celery juice can be helpful.

2. Food that Heal: Dark Chocolate, Peanut Butter, Lettuce, Cucumber, Sunflower seeds, Yogurt and Tomato are also helpful. **Garlic** is useful to lower the blood high cholesterol by the scientific research. **Pomegranate, Ginger, Almonds** and **Walnuts** and **Grape Seed Extract are well known by their effects on improving heart functions.**

3. Herbs that Heal: Eating 1 tsp of flax seed and black seed every morning for 3 months is good for heart. They also cure high cholesterol and triglycerides due to obesity, as both seeds have weight reducing properties. The Indian herb; Guggul and Hawthorne are the best herbs for heart.

4. Milk that Heals: Camel milk (as narrated by Prophet Mohammad (PBUH) offers endless health benefits. One of those is treating heart problems. Camel milk is said to be the vasodilator of the Future". My patients who took 2 glasses of camel milk daily or our food supplement: **Heart Life** for 3 months found miracle results for both heart and sex!!!!!

5. Herbal Tea that Heals: Hundreds of heart cases who took our herbal tea ;**Heart & Love Tea** which is simply composed of Cinnamon, Fenugreek and **Coriander seed** for 3-6 months could easily improve heart functions without medications!!!!!

6. Food Supplemnts that Heal: Many patients obtained excellent results by using our food supplement named: **Heart Life** which contains a number of anti-lipid herbs including **Coriander seed!!!!**

A recent experiment from the Biochemistry Department at the University of Kerala, in India, studied the effects of coriander seeds on rats that had been fed a very high-fat, high-cholesterol diet. Researchers saw significant drops in total cholesterol and triglyceride levels in the rats and their hearts became more healthy.

CORIANDER AND HEMORROHIDS

25% of all adults suffer from hemorrhoids at some time in their lives. Hemorrhoids are dilated, stretched, or swollen veins that appear in or around the rectal opening. There may be blood dots within the veins, and sometimes hemorrhoids protrude out of the rectum. They may itch, tear, bleed, and cause extreme pain. In some cases, blood may be visible on the surface of the stools or on toilet paper. Poor circulation and weakness of the blood vessels contribute to hemorrhoids. Straining during bowel movements can aggravate hemorrhoids or lead to their development. Other contributing factors include allergies, recurrent constipation, lack of exercise, lifting heavy objects, obesity, poor nutrition, and standing or sitting for long periods of time. Pregnant women often get hemorrhoids as a result of the added pressure and weight on their pelvic veins.

How to Rid Hemorrhoids in 4 Weeks without Medications which will be printed in the United States soon.

We can draw the main guidelines of our protocol as follows:

1. Juice that Heal: Add dry ginger powder in buttermilk and drink it to cure piles-wart. Soak coriander seeds in water at night, in the morning mash it; drink that water or otherwise coriander juice to stop the blood falling from the wart. Blood falling from the wart is stopped by drinking the decoction of **coriander seed** and sugar. By drinking 1-2 tsp of castor oil along with hot milk relieves pain caused due to piles and also avoids scratches on the anus.

2. Food that Heal: Piles-Wart is cured by eating grinded sesame in butter, In the morning when the stomach is empty, take a handful of black sesame, chew it and eat it along with sugar to stop the blood falling from the piles Piles-Wart is cured by taking mango seed powder along with honey, **Baking Powder are well known by their effects on improving** piles. Cut onions in to small pieces and dry it in the sun, take little pieces of onion, fry it in the ghee, add little black sesame and sugar powder and eat it in the morning to cure wart. Figs, Apricots are important fruits.

3. Herbs that Heal: Roast black cumin seeds; add equal proportion of black pepper and rock salt in it to make a powder. Intake this powder along with butter milk after meal to cure piles-wart. Grind **coriander**, heat it, make a bundle and foment with it to relieve the pain caused due to wart. A wart is cured by in taking finely filtered pure turmeric powder along with water before sleeping at night.

4. Milk that Heals: Camel milk (as narrated by Prophet Mohammad (PBUH) offers endless health benefits. One of those is treating piles. My patients who took 2 glasses of camel milk daily for 4 weeks found miracle results for both piles and sex!!!!!

5. Herbal Tea that Heals: Hundreds of piles cases who took our herbal tea ;Diges Tech Tea which is simply composed of Chamomile, Oak Bark, Propolis and **Coriander** seed for 3 weeks could easily solve their piles without medications!!!

6. Food Supplemnts that Heal: Many patients obtained excellent results by using our food supplement named: Hemo

Tech together with our cream: **Hemo Tech Cream**. Piles are cured by eating mangos teen ketchup along with milk cream.

7. Bath that Heals: 2 drops cypress oil, 2 drops juniper oil. Add the cypress and juniper oils to a shallow tub filled with warm water. Sit hip-deep in the bath for twenty minutes. Another very successful bath my patients used and it did work for years: Equal parts of Oak Leaf, Oak Fruit Peel, Oak Bark and Chamomile are boiled in water bath for 20 minutes and used by sitting anus on it directly for 10 minutes twice daily for 2 weeks only!!!!!

8. Essential Oils that Heals:

1 ounce jojoba oil 4 drops cypress oil 4 drops tea tree oil
3 drops **coriander oil**
3 drops myrrh oil

Place the jojoba oil in a clean container, add the essential oils, and gently turn the container upside down several times or roll it between your hands to blend. Apply the oil externally, as needed.

CORIANDER AND HYPERTENSION

A rise in blood pressure above the normal is referred to as high blood pressure or hypertension. But what is blood pressure?

Blood pressure is determined by the force of the contraction of the heart muscle, the resistance or elasticity of the vessel wall, the quantity of blood being pumped from the heart into the vessels, and lastly the viscosity of the blood. The latter depends upon the cellular or fluid constituents which make up the blood volume.

What are the Causes and Symptoms of Hypertension?

A faulty diet, smoking, negative emotional feelings, anxiety and stress are factors which often have a direct bearing on blood pressure. The elasticity of the blood-vessel walls diminishes with age, and certain deposits accumulate on the inner lining. For some reasons, some people are genetically predisposed to this condition. They have a familial tendency to certain lipid (fat) metabolic disorders.

High blood pressure in the early stages usually goes undetected. It is often an accidental finding during a medical check-up for other reasons. However, headaches, fatigue, nosebleeds, shortness of breath, swelling of the feet, palpitations, and nervousness are symptoms that warrant the necessity of an early blood-pressure check-up. In the early stages the high blood pressure have no symptoms.

From the phytochemical composition of coriander we can notice a number of chemical compounds forming Coriander act as anti-stress hypotensive vasodilator agents, which clearly means that coriander is a good candidate to be safely used for hypertension (high blood pressure).

Coriander serves both as an herb and a spice. It is a healing herb that is used effectively in different parts of the globe. While Indians use it for its anti-inflammatory properties, many other nations use this perennial herb for **diuretic** and carminative qualities for **hypertension**.

In for hypertension management it has been shown that Coriander acts as an anti-stress hypotensive agent and also helps in the vasodilation of veins!!

Many hypertensive cases used **Coriander seed tea** from kitchen together with my powerful **PRESS OIL** which is used externally 5 times a day as a relaxing agent. All cases including myself got rid of high blood pressure for good in less than 24 weeks!!!! I discovered myself with high blood pressure of 190/105 3 years ago and I started taking my relaxation oil (PRESS OIL) together with coriander tea and after 12 weeks only I measured my blood pressure and found it normal!!!!!Now my pressure reads 120/80 and sometimes 110/70 without any medications!!!!!

Natural Methods of Treating Hypertension:

You can find full details of our natural protocol of treating hypertension in our book:

How to Lower Your High Blood Pressure to Normal without Medications which will be printed in the United States soon.

We can draw the main guidelines of our protocol as follows:

1. Juice that Heal: Noni, Tomato, Cucumber, and Celery juice can be helpful.

2. Food that Heal: Banana and Potato (rich in potassium), Cocoa, Dark Chocolate, Brown Algae, Lettuce, Cucumber, Yogurt and Tomato are also helpful... Garlic is useful to lower the blood pressure by the scientific research.

3. Herbs that Heal: Eating 1 tsp of khella and flax seed every morning for 3 months is said to prevent hypertension due to heredity factors. They also cure hypertension due to obesity, as both seeds have weight reducing properties.

4. Milk that Heals: Camel milk (as narrated by Prophet Mohammad (PBUH) offers endless health benefits. One of those is treating hypertension. Camel milk is said to be the vasodilator of the Future". My patients who took 2 glasses of camel milk daily or our food supplement: **Camel Tech** for 3 months found miracle results for both hypertension and sex!!!!!

5. Herbal Tea that Heals: Hundreds of hypertensives who took our herbal tea ;**Relax Tea** which is simply composed of Hibiscus, Olive Leaf, Linden and **Coriander seed** for 3-6 months could easily reduce their high blood pressure to normal without medications!!!!!

6. Food Supplemnts that Heal: Many patients obtained excellent results by using our food supplement named: **Press Tech** which contains a number of hypotensive herbs including **Coriander seed!!!!**

7. Essential Oils that Heal: Our oil mix; Press Oil was successfully used with hundreds of hypertensive patients together with Coriander tea and all of them became hypertension free!!!!!!

8. Sex that Heals: It was found by a number of researchers that performing sex 3 times weekly reduces and may cure blood pressure permanently!!!!!

9. Water that Heals: Honey Water

It is narrated in QURAN that honey is a complete cure!!! I supervised a graduate student who tested using water and different percentages of honey in capillary tubes similar to veins and we published our findings in the International J.Biomedical Engineering 10 years ago!!!! The results of study showed that a Drinking honey water: a mixture of 1 tbs of honey in a glass of water reduces blood pressure, cholesterol and maintains vasodilatation.!!!!!!!!

Pulmonary Hypertension:

Pulmonary hypertension is a very difficult condition everywhere in the world and it is well known that nobody arrived at a cure!!!!! By using our natural protocol for hypertension a number of severe cases; one of them is a medical doctor solved their pulmonary hypertension for good!!!!! And he sent me a letter of acknowledgement!!!!!!

CORIANDER AND INSOMNIA

Insomnia is a sleeping disorder characterized by persistent difficulty falling asleep or staying asleep despite the opportunity. It is typically followed by functional impairment while awake. Insomniacs have been known to complain about being unable to close their eyes or "rest their mind" for more than a few minutes at a time. Both organic and non-organic insomnia constitute a sleep disorder

For Sleep Disorder (Insomnia): Paste of coriander leaves should be applied on forehead to induce sleep or else, take orally fresh juice of leaves with some sugar-candy.

Coriander has been used as a folk medicine for the relief of anxiety and insomnia in Iranian folk medicine. Experiments in mice support its use as an anxiolytic.

Insomnia Home Remedy Using Gotu kola Coriander Cumin and Water Spinach:

How to use it:

Take 1 spoon of cumin seeds, 3 stalks of water spinach, 2 pegagan leaves, and 1/4 tsp coriander. Boil the whole ingredients with 2 glass of water until there is only 1 glass left of it. Then put it through a sieve and drink it before sleep. Do it every day until the desired results are achieved.

Natural Methods of Treating Insomnia:

You can find full details of our natural protocol of treating high insomnia in our book:

Solve Your Insomnia in 4 Weeks without Medications which will be printed in the United States soon.

We can draw the main guidelines of our protocol as follows:

1. Juice that Heal: Lemon-Lemon Balm juice can be very helpful.

2. Foods that Heal: Whole Lemon

3. Herbs that Heal: Hops, Chamomile, Lemon Balm, Valerian and Passion Flower.

4.Herbal Tea that Heals: Hundreds of insomnia cases who took our herbal tea ;**Relax U Tea** which is simply composed of Lemon Balm, Chamomile and **Coriander seed** for weeks could easily solve their insomnia without medications!!

CORIANDER AND IRRITABLE COLON

(IRRITABLE BOWEL SYNDROME –IBS)

Coriander Seed is considered a carminative that will help prevent gas from forming in the intestines and will also help expel wind from the bowels. In addition, Coriander is believed to allay the "griping" (pain and grumbling in the bowels) often associated with other laxatives.

As an antispasmodic, Coriander is thought to help relieve diarrhea and ease abdominal cramps.

Coriander contains substances that are antibacterial and antifungal, helping to prevent infections from developing in wounds. Topically applied, the essential oil in Coriander has been used to ease the pain of rheumatic joints, sore muscles, neuralgia and sciatica, which appear to attest to its anti-inflammatory reputation.

COLON AND GASES:

Cure a cranky irritable digestion this way:
Stress hits women in the digestive tract. During high-stress times reach for these herbs and spices:
Cilantro tones up your digestion.
Coriander seeds ease gas.
Cardamom reduces mucous-forming effects of dairy foods.
Turmeric helps your liver work more efficiently.
Black pepper helps you digest dairy foods.
Fennel prevents gas.

Coriander serves both as an herb and a spice. It is a healing herb that is used effectively in different parts of the globe. While Indians use it for its anti-inflammatory properties, many other nations use this herb for digestion.

We have many successful stories about using **coriander** seed tea for irritable colon!!

Natural Methods of Treating Irritable Colon:

You can find full details of our natural protocol of treating irritable colon problems in our book:

The Only Fast Cure for Irritable Colon in the World which will be printed in the United States soon.

We can draw the main guidelines of our protocol as follows:

1. Juice that Heal: Wheatgrass, Mint-Lemon juice can be very helpful.

2. Food that Heal: Propolis and Licorice are useful to solve irritable colon problems by the scientific research.

3. Herbs that Heal: Eating 1 tsp of Caraway, Fennel, and Anise every morning for 3 months is good for irritable colon.

4. Milk that Heals: Camel milk (as narrated by Prophet Mohammad (PBUH) offers endless health benefits. One of those is treating irritable colon. My patients who took 2 glasses of camel milk daily for 3 months found miracle results for both irritable colon and sex!!!!!

5. Herbal Tea that Heals: Hundreds of irritable colon cases who took our herbal tea; Diges **Tech Tea** which is simply composed of Mint, Fennel, Anise, and **Coriander seed** for 3 months could easily solve their irritable colon problem without medications!!!!!

CORIANDER AND JAUNDICE

Jaundice is a condition characterized by the yellowing of the whites of the eyes, the mucous membranes, urine and the <u>skin</u>. It is often caused by dysfunction of the liver. The yellow coloring comes from bilirubin, which is caused by aging red blood cells. The accumulation of excessive red blood cells within the body results in jaundice.

As for drinks, one should avoid alcoholic drinks completely.

From the phytochemical composition of coriander we can notice a number of chemical compounds forming Coriander act as excellent an anti-inflammatory agent, which clearly means that coriander is a good candidate to be safely used for jaundice!!!.

Coriander seeds also can help cure jaundice by reducing yellowness of the skin and whites of the eyes.

Natural Methods of Treating Jaundice Problems:

You can find full details of our natural protocol of treating jaundice problems in our book:

How to Rid Jaundice in 3 Days without Medications which will be printed in the United States soon.

We can draw the main guidelines of our protocol as follows:

1. Juice that Heal: Lemon JUICE, One glass of sugar cane juice, mixed with the juice of half a lime, and taken twice daily, can hasten recovery from jaundice and Tomato juice and Barley water drink can be very helpful.

2. Food that Heal: Honey, Lemon, Cucumber, Cabbage and Tomato are also helpful... Pomegranate, Almonds, Dried Dates and Cardamoms, **Baking Powder are well known by their effects on** jaundice. The green leaves of radish are another valuable remedy for jaundice

3. Herbs that Heal: Eating 1 tsp of cinnamon and black seed with honey every morning for 2 weeks is good for jaundice. The Indian herb; Shilajit is one of the best herbs for jaundice. Milk Thistle, Dandelion and **Andrographis are also very useful.**

4. Milk that Heals: Camel milk (as narrated by Prophet Mohammad (PBUH) offers endless health benefits. One of those is treating jaundice problems. My patients who took 2 glasses of camel milk daily or our food supplement **Liv Tech** for 2 weeks found miracle results for both jaundice and sex!!!!!

5. Herbal Tea that Heals: Hundreds of jaundice cases who took our herbal tea ;**Liv Tea** which is simply composed of Radish Leaf, Lemon Balm and **Coriander** seed for 2 weeks could easily solve their jaundice problem without medications.

6. Food Supplemnts that Heal: Many patients obtained excellent results by using our food supplement named: **Liv Tech** which contains a number of anti-inflammatory herbs including **Coriander** seed!! Together with chlorophyll supplement.

7. Avoid: Smoking and Drinking Alcohol.

CORIANDER AND KIDNEY HEALTH

In renal failure the kidneys undergo cellular death and are unable to filter wastes, produce urine and maintain fluid balances. This dysfunction causes a buildup of toxins in the body which can affect the blood, brain and heart, as well as other complications. Renal failure is very serious and even deadly if left untreated.

The symptoms of renal failure include edema, which is an accumulation of fluid characterized by swelling, and a decrease in urination. Other symptoms may include a general ill feeling, exhaustion and headaches. Often, a person with renal failure does not experience any symptoms

From the phytochemical composition of coriander we can notice a number of chemical compounds forming Coriander act as excellent **diuretic** anti-edema agents, which clearly means that coriander is a good candidate to be safely used for renal(kidney)failure!!!.

Coriander serves both as an herb and a spice. It is a healing herb that is used effectively in different parts of the globe. While Indians use it for its anti-inflammatory properties, many other nations use this perennial herb for kidney health.

Many stories about using coriander seed tea as a diuretic and carminative tool for hypertension (high blood pressure) and for **renal (kidney) failure!!!!** Two Qatari patients with renal failure; one was on dialysis and the other was about to start dialysis: both avoided dialysis after starting taking **coriander tea** together with our food supplement **RENO**

TECH and asparagus soup!!!Many other patients avoided or stopped dialysis after following our nutrition protocol.

Many kidney cases used **Coriander seed tea** from kitchen together with my powerful **Reno Tech** food supplement and after 3 months they got excellent results without any medications!!!!!

Natural Methods of Treating Heart Problems:

You can find full details of our natural protocol of treating kidney problems in our book:

How to Avoid Dialysis without Medications which will be printed in the United States soon.

We can draw the main guidelines of our protocol as follows:

1. Juice that Heal: Noni, Tomato, **Cranberry**, Aoe Vera and Celery juice can be helpful.

2. Food that Heal: Asparagus Soup, Lettuce, Cucumber, Cabbage and Tomato are also helpful. **Garlic** is useful to lower the blood pressure and improve kidney function by the scientific research. **Pomegranate, Ginger, Almonds** and **Walnuts** and **Grape Seed Extract, Baking Powder is well known by their effects on improving kidney functions.**

3. Herbs that Heal: Eating 1 tsp of flax seed and black seed every morning for 3 months is good for kidney. The Indian herb; Shilajit is one of the best herbs for kidney. **Dandelion and Tribulus terrestris are also very useful.**

4. Milk that Heals: Camel milk (as narrated by Prophet Mohammad (PBUH) offers endless health benefits. One of those is treating kidney problems. My patients who took 2 glasses of camel milk daily or our food supplement **Reno**

Tech for 3 months found miracle results for both kidney and sex!!!!!

5. Herbal Tea that Heals: Hundreds of kidney cases who took our herbal tea ;**Press Tea** which is simply composed of Celery, Linden and **Coriander seed** for 3-6 months could easily improve heart functions without medications!!!!!

6. Food Supplemnts that Heal: Many patients obtained excellent results by using our food supplement named: **Reno Tech** which contains a number of **diuretic** herbs including **Coriander seed!!!!**Together with **chlorophyll** supplement.

CORIANDER AND LIVER CIRRHOSIS

Cirrhosis is a complication of many liver diseases that is characterized by abnormal structure and function of the liver. The diseases that lead to cirrhosis do so because they injure and kill liver cells and the inflammation and repair that is associated with the dying liver cells causes scar tissue to form. The liver cells that do not die multiply in an attempt to replace the cells that have died. This results in clusters of newly-formed liver cells (regenerative nodules) within the scar tissue. There are many causes of cirrhosis; they include chemicals (such as alcohol, Qat consumption(in Yemen), fat, and certain medications), viruses, toxic metals (such as iron and copper that accumulate in the liver as a result of genetic diseases), and autoimmune liver disease in which the body's immune system attacks the liver.

Enlarged Liver:

The liver is one of the largest organs in the body. Its functions include filtering the blood, producing bile and amino acids, and serving as a storage site for glucose. When the liver becomes enlarged or "fatty," the body can suffer serious side effects, some of which can be fatal if left untreated. Here are some of the factors that cause hepatomegaly, or enlargement of the liver:

Congestive Heart Failure, Alcohol, Hemochromatosis which is a condition wherein there is an excessive amount of iron in the body, **Cancer, Hepatitis, Nonalcoholic fatty liver disease**, seen in people with obesity, diabetes or high cholesterol, causes an accumulation of fat in the liver. The result is inflammation and subsequent enlargement of the liver.

People with liver problems should not take alcohol at all. A healthy diet with fruits and vegetables is advised.

Coriander can help fortifying the liver. You will need 1.5 teaspoons of coriander seeds. Add a cup of boiling water. Repeat it 3 times daily.

You can take the food supplements: **Liv Tech** and **Liv52**.

Natural Methods of Treating Liver Problems:

You can find full details of our natural protocol of treating liver problems in our book: **How to Fix Your Liver without Medications** which will be printed in the United States soon.

We can draw the main guidelines of our protocol as follows:

1. Juice that Heal: White Radish, Wheatgrass, Cucumber, and Celery juice can be helpful.

2. Food that Heal:, Lettuce, Cucumber, Yogurt and Tomato are also helpful. Pomegranate, Ginger, Almonds and **Grape Seed Extract are well known by their effects on improving liver functions.**

3. Herbs that Heal: Eating 1 tsp of coriander seed and black seed with honey every morning for 3 months is good for liver.

4. Milk that Heals: Camel milk mixed with camel urine (as narrated by Prophet Mohammad (PBUH) offers endless health benefits. One of those is treating liver problems: Cirrhosis, Enlargement, Hepatitis B & C ad Liver Cancer. Camel milk is said to be the **Liver Cure of the Future**". My patients who took 2 glasses of camel milk (mixed with camel urine) daily or our food supplement: **Camel Tech for** 3-6 months found miracle results for both liver and sex!!!!!

5. Herbal Tea that Heals: Hundreds of liver cases who took our herbal tea ;**Liv & Love Tea** which is simply composed of Cinnamon, Fenugreek and **Coriander seed** for 3-6 months could easily improve liver functions without medications!!!!!

6. Food Supplemnts that Heal: Many patients obtained excellent results by using our food supplement named: **Camel Life** which contains a number of anti-cirrhotic herbs including **Coriander** seed together with chlorophyll food supplement.

A recent experiment from the Biology Department at the University of King Abdul Aziz in Saudi, on rats showed excellent results on immune system and cancer.

Liver Detox Secret! Turmeric and Coriander Heal Liver!

It is well known that liver represents the filter and port that receives all toxins from other parts of the body and when it is overloaded by toxins of food, drugs or chemotherapy sources it does need a process of detoxification by certain types of herbs; one of them is **Coriander.**

For example the following procedure is given by one of the experts asked about the detox process after chemotherapy and this process can be followed by any person at many stations in his life:

By Nancy Lonsdorf, MD:

Q. Over the past few years, I've had surgery and chemo for cancer. How can I restore my immune and hormonal

systems?

A. Although most of the effects of chemotherapy are short-term, some—including fatigue, impaired immunity, hormonal imbalances, and temporary problems with memory, attention, and concentration (recently dubbed "chemobrain")—can persist for years. To date, not many researchers have looked at the efficacy of treatments to reverse or prevent these long-term side effects. However, it makes sense that approaches that support detoxification reduce stress, and rebuild immunity will help speed your recovery from both the cancer and its treatment.

Reducing damage to the body during treatment also may prevent side effects down the line. In laboratory studies, researchers found that one traditional Ayurvedic herbal formula called amrit nectar protects normal cells from chemotherapy injury. In another small clinical trial, the formula reduced side effects and improved overall strength and well-being without interfering with chemo's anti-cancer effects. My clinical experience with traditional detoxification approaches from ayurveda, the traditional health system of India, has convinced me that cleansing the body of toxins and rebalancing the body after cancer treatment can help restore optimum health. This type of ayurvedic detox has two phases. Phase I: During the first eight weeks when your body is recovering strength and stamina, eat a wholesome diet with immune-boosting herbs and spices, drink plenty of pure water, reduce stress, and get extra sleep to enhance your body's own healing response.

Follow the tips below for optimal detox and recovery during this time.

• Eat organically grown foods, including whole grains, legumes, unprocessed nuts and seeds, and seven to 10 servings of fresh vegetables, fruits, and freshly squeezed juices each day.

• Avoid alcohol, refined sugar, artificial ingredients, cigarette smoke, chemicals, and pollution.

• Cook with turmeric, coriander, cilantro, basil, oregano, rosemary, ginger, garlic, cinnamon, fennel, clove, and saffron to support immunity, hormonal balance, detoxification, and antioxidant protection.

• Take soluble fiber such as psyllium husks to promote elimination of toxins excreted by the liver via the stool.
• Drink eight glasses of warm, pure spring water daily.
• Lower your stress with effective techniques such as yoga and meditation. Research has shown that Transcendental Meditation enhances quality of life in breast cancer patients, reduces stress hormone levels, promotes longevity, and boosts DNA repair.

• Support liver detox and the production of glutathione, the body's primary defense against most toxins, with plenty of protein in your diet. No vegetarians are advised to favor more easily digestible sources such as organic poultry and wild-caught fish that are low in mercury. Vegetarians may wish to include organic, high-protein vegetable sources such as soaked nuts and seeds, legumes, quinoa, amaranth, spirulina, and hemp-seed nut. Consult your doctor before increasing soy in your   diet.
• Drink this simple detox tea to support liver and kidney function: Add 1/4 teaspoon whole cumin seed, 1/2 teaspoon whole coriander, and 1/4 teaspoon whole fennel to two quarts

of boiled hot, pure spring water; let steep, and sip throughout the day for two months.

Phase II: After two months, if you still feel in need of detox, consider the intensive level of Ayurvedic detox called panchakarma, traditionally done in-residence under professional supervision.

Check out The Raj (www.theraj.com), a health spa offering holistic and natural maharishi ayurveda treatments and massage. Panchakarma includes warm oil massages, gentle heat treatments, and mild elimination therapies to remove both water- and fat-soluble toxins from deep in the tissues. (Other non-Ayurvedic detoxification approaches, such as steam baths, saunas, aerobic exercise, and drinking large amounts of water, can also reduce water-soluble toxins substantially.) In one two-month study, five days of panchakarma treatments resulted in a 46 percent drop in blood levels of PCBs and 58 percent drop in beta-HCH, prevalent environmental toxins linked to cancer and other serious disorders. It is always best to detox under professional supervision with methods supported by research and an established safety track record.

CORIANDER AND LOST APPETITE

A sign of good health is the presence of a healthy appetite-a good appetite will be neither over powering nor very mild in the way it affects the person. The fact is that even the slightest physical or emotional problems can affect the appetite of a person, and for this reason the presence of a poor appetite may not necessarily be a major health concern. Appetite problems can come in different ways and some other physical symptoms of a malfunctioning appetite include the presence of abdominal bloating, persistent <u>indigestion</u> and <u>constipation</u> - sensations of <u>nausea</u> or <u>pain</u> can also be felt if the appetite is affected in some cases. The cause of the drop in appetite will brook further investigation when the sudden or gradual appetite loss comes along with any kind of <u>weight loss</u> - a medical examination becomes important in such cases as it could be a signal for the presence of some other serious disorder - a poor appetite can then be a symptom for an underlying condition.

Coriander is a great herbal remedy for restoring lost appetite.

1. Juice that Heal: Wheatgrass, Mint-Lemon juice can be very helpful.

2. Food that Heal: Okra is also helpful. Propolis and Licorice are useful to solve digestion problems by the scientific research.

3. Herbs that Heal: Alfalfa, Lemon Balm, Mint, Ginger, Cardamom, Wormwood.

4. Milk that Heals: Camel milk (as narrated by Prophet Mohammad (PBUH) offers endless health benefits. One of those is treating Appetite problems. My patients who took 2 glasses of camel milk daily for 3 weeks found miracle results for both Appetite and sex!!!!!

5. Herbal Tea that Heals: Many cases who took our herbal tea; Diges Tech Tea which is simply composed of Mint, Ginger, Lemon Balm and **Coriander** seed for 3 weeks could easily solve their Appetite problem without medications!!

6. Vitamins that Heal-Complex, Folic Acid, Zinc.

7. Essential Oils that Heal: Commonly used essential oils for appetite loss:

Bergamot, Caraway, Chamomile, Cinnamon, Coriander, Ginger, Hyssop, Ylang Ylang.

CORIANDER AND MEMORY

It is well known that **coriander** improved blood circulation throughout the body and hence improves memory.

We used coriander seed together with black seed, gotu kola and ginkgo biloba as an herbal tea on a number of students and all of them showed improvement in memory, vitality and clear way of thinking!!!

We also used coriander oil mixed with brahmi oil, rosemary oil and ginger oil on another number of students on their face foreheads and all of them showed an excellent progress in their school!!!

The tea mentioned above was used as a fruit drink mixed with cranberry/strawberry juices and the results were the same.

Other good home remedies to improve memory are:

Milk and honey have been shown to help improve your memory. While there are many books you can buy which will present a number of techniques you can use to improve your memory.

Also Almond and almond milk. Fish oil, Walnut, Rosemary, Ginseng, and Pistachio are very useful for memory.

CORIANDER AND MENSTRUAL FLOW PROBLEMS

Heavy menstrual bleeding and clotting are common problems for many women. When a woman soaks a pad or a tampon an hour for several hours or more or bleeds for more than a week and a half each month, this is called *menorrhagia*. If she soaks through two or more pads or tampons an hour, this is generally considered *hypermenorrhagia*

Coriander seeds check excessive menstrual flow. 6 grams of the seeds should be boiled in half a liter of water, till only half the water remains. Sugar or honey should be added to it and taken when it is still warm. The patient gets relief after taking this for 3 or 4 days.

Other Home Remedies for Menstruation:

Menstruation treatment with Parsley: Parsley is one of the most efficient among the several home remedies in the treatment of menstrual disorders. It increases menstruation and helps in the regularization of the monthly periods.

Menstruation treatment with Ginger: The use of ginger is a useful home remedy for menstrual disorders, especially in cases of painful menstruation and stoppage of menstrual flow.

Menstruation treatment with Sesame Seeds: Sesame seeds are precious in Menstruation. Half a teaspoon of powder of these seeds, taken with hot water two times daily, acts brilliantly in reducing spasmodic pain during menstruation in young, unmarried anemic girls.

Menstruation treatment via Papaya: The unripe papaya helps the contractions of the muscle fibers of the uterus and is thus helpful in securing a proper menstrual flow. Papaya is especially useful when menstruation ceases due to stress or fright in young unmarried girls.

Menstruation treatment with Marigold: The herb Marigold, named after the Virgin Mary, is helpful in allaying any pain during menstruation and smoothes the progress of menstrual flow. An infusion of the herb must be given in doses of one tablespoon two times every day for the treatment of these disorders.

Menstruation treatment with Banana Flower: The use of banana flower is one of the most efficient home remedies in the treatment of menorrhagia or excessive menstruation. One banana flower should be cooked and consumed with one cup of curd. This will increase the quantity of progesterone and decrease the bleeding.

Menstruation treatment with Mango Bark: The juice of the fresh mango bark is one more valuable remedy for heavy bleeding during menstruation. The juice is given with the addition of white of an egg as an option, a mixture of 10 ml of a fluid extract of the bark, and 120 ml of water may be given in doses of one teaspoon every hour or two.

Menstruation treatment with Barberry: The herb Indian barberry is helpful in case of excessive bleeding. It should be given in doses of 13-25 grams every day.

Menstruation treatment with Hermal: Hermal is useful in regulating the menstrual periods. It is particularly beneficial in painful and difficult menstruation. Two tablespoons of the seeds should be boiled in half a liter of water, till it is decreased by one - third. This decoction should be prearranged in 15 to 3 0ml doses.

CORIANDER AND MOUTH ULCER

Mouth ulcer is the loss of delicate tissue that lines inside the mouth caused by a break in the mucous membrane or epithelium on the lips.

What Causes Mouth Ulcers?

Among the factors causing mouth ulcer are stress, fatigue, illness, injury from accidental biting, hormonal changes, burns from eating hot food, poor oral hygiene, menstruation, sudden weight loss, food allergies, deficiencies in vitamin B12, iron and folic acid, certain drugs, chemicals. In some cases, mouth ulcers are not harmful and resolve by themselves in a few days without any treatment.

• Infection with a type of bacteria called Helicobacter pylori (**H. pylori**) also causes mouth ulcer.

• Use of painkillers called nonsteroidal anti-inflammatory drugs (NSAIDs), such as aspirin, naproxen (Aleve, Anaprox, Naprosyn, and others), ibuprofen (Motrin, Advil, Midol, and others), and many others available by prescription. Even aspirin coated with a special substance can still cause ulcers.

• Excess acid production from gastronomes, tumors of the acid producing cells of the stomach that increases acid output.

Coriander helps cure mouth ulcer, inflammation and spasm.

Diet for Mouth Ulcers

Whenever mouth ulcers occur avoid hot, spicy food, caffeine and tea. Consume green vegetables as much as possible as green vegetables provide the necessary fibber for the movement of bowels which prevents constipation, advisable to stop fatty food. Papaya is a very good fruit to be consumed in mouth ulcers. It soothes the mouth ulcers and helps in quick recovery.

Home Cure:

Paste of garlic in coconut milk is useful in mouth ulcer, Chew holy basil leaf, Apply milk of raw papaya on ulcer, **Gargle with coriander seed boil water,** Paste of Indian plum leaves

As for drinks, one should avoid alcoholic drinks completely during mouth ulcer attack.

Coriander serves both as an herb and a spice. It is a healing herb that is used effectively in different parts of the globe. While Indians use it for its anti-inflammatory properties, many other nations use this perennial herb for mouth ulcer.

Natural Methods of Treating Mouth Ulcer:

You can find full details of our natural protocol of treating gout problems in our book: **How to Fix Mouth Ulcer without Medications** which will be printed in the United States soon.

We can draw the main guidelines of our protocol as follows:

1. Juice that Heal: Licorice, Cabbage juice can be very helpful.

2. Food that Heal: Cherry, Lettuce, Cucumber, Cabbage are also helpful. Pomegranate, Ginger, Almonds, Walnuts, **Baking Powder are well known by their effects on improving** mouth ulcer.

3. Herbs that Heal: Eating 1 tsp of Fenugreek, Aloe Vera, Ginger, Lemon Balm, Chamomile, Peppermint, Licorice and black seed every morning for 3 weeks is good for mouth ulcer. The Indian herb; Shilajit is one of the best herbs for mouth ulcer.

4. Milk that Heals: Camel milk (as narrated by Prophet Mohammad (PBUH) offers endless health benefits. One of those is treating mouth ulcer. My patients who took 2 glasses of camel milk daily for 3 months found miracle results for both mouth ulcer and sex!!!!!

5. Herbal Tea that Heals: Hundreds of mouth ulcer cases who took our herbal tea ;**Diges Tech Tea** which is simply composed of Licorice, Alfalfa, Pomegranate Peels, Propolis and **Coriander seed** for 3 weeks could easily solve their mouth ulcer problem without medications!!!!!

6. Food Supplemnts that Heal: Many patients obtained excellent results by using our food supplement named: **Stomach Care** which contains a number of herbs including **Coriander seed!!!!**Together with **chlorophyll** supplement.

7. Essential Oils that Heal: Citronelol, a component of essential oils in **coriander**, is an excellent antiseptic. In addition, other components have anti microbial and healing effects which do not let wounds and ulcers in the mouth go worse. They aid healing up of ulcers and freshen up the breath

CORIANDER AND NOSE BLEED

Nose Bleed is a common condition which one sees especially in children. Nose Bleed is also known as Epistaxis and Bleeding from the nose. The blood vessels in the nasal passage are very tender and easily rupture with the slightest pressure or injury. Since the veins of the nose are devoid of valves therefore the bleeding is usually very heavy. Coriander leaves extract is very beneficial in resolving the incidence of Nose Bleed.

As one of the home remedies for nosebleed, you can add a piece of camphor in small amounts of **coriander** leaves. The Nose Bleed is resolved immediately with the medicinal benefits of **Coriander** leaves.

Here are some of the Common Home Remedies for the Treatment of Nose Bleeding:

Coriander Leaves - Use juice of fresh coriander leaves as nasal drops.

Alum - Herbalists suggest using wild alum root powder. This will stop the bleeding immediately. Wild alum root is a powerful astringent.

Lemon Juice - Mix the juice of three lemons into two cups of cold water and sponge on the sunburn. The lemon will cool the burn, act as a disinfectant, and will promote healing of the skin.

Goldenseal - This one is another good remedy used for curing nose bleeds. Make a tea from goldenseal using one teaspoon to a pint of boiling water. Steep a few minutes and let it settle at the bottom, and when it is cooled down - snuff some into your nostrils. Do this several times during the day to prevent recurrence.

Tulsi Juice - Drinking tulsi juice mixed with honey will also help and provide extra strength to the body.

Vinegar - Pour some vinegar on a cloth and wash the neck, nose and temples with it

CORIANDER AND ODEMA (SWELLING)

Edema also known as odema means swelling of body parts due to fluid retention. It is the accumulation of excessive serous fluids in cells or cavities of the body. It mainly affects lower body parts, mostly foot and ankles. It can slow down the healing process, increase the chances of developing skin infection, affect blood circulation and can be painful. Edema is not a disease; it only indicates that something is wrong in the body. Edema is due to an underlying problem in the body. It usually occurs in the feet, ankles and legs, but it can involve your entire body.

Causes of edema include:

Eating too much salt, Sunburn, <u>Heart failure</u>, <u>Kidney disease</u>, Liver problems from <u>cirrhosis</u>, Pregnancy, Problems with <u>lymph nodes</u>, especially after <u>mastectomy</u>, Some medicines, Standing or walking a lot when the weather is warm

The symptoms of renal failure include <u>edema</u>, which is an accumulation of fluid characterized by swelling, and a decrease in urination. Other symptoms may include a general ill feeling, exhaustion and headaches. Often, a person with renal failure does not experience any symptoms

From the phytochemical composition of coriander we can notice a number of chemical compounds forming Coriander act as excellent **diuretic** anti-edema agents, which clearly means that coriander is a good candidate to be safely used for odema swelling of any kind!!!.

Coriander seeds can help the body in flushing out excess fluids.

Coriander serves both as an herb and a spice. It is a healing herb that is used effectively in different parts of the globe. While Indians use it for its anti-inflammatory properties, many other nations use this perennial herb for odema.

Many stories about using coriander seed tea as a diuretic tool for getting rid of odema and swelling. One of them was my favorite patient Mrs. Aisha Khulaifi from Qatar who suddenly suffered from foot swelling and could not wear her shoes!!!!Mrs. Aisha is a highly educated pleasant woman who believes in natural alternative solutions for all human health problems and she together with her big family got beautiful results after they used our natural formulas for different disorders!!!! She called me when I was on my way from Amman to Dubai asking about fast solution for her foot. I asked her to use coriander seed tea 2 to 3 times daily for 3 days!

She called me the second day full of joy and said" **Iam flying in the sky!!!!!**" My foot problem has been solved fast and I am able to wear my shoes easily in less than 24 hours!!!!!!

Many kidney cases used **Coriander seed tea** from kitchen together with my powerful **Reno Tech** food supplement and after 3 months they got excellent results without any medications!!!!!

Natural Methods of Treating Odema and Swelling:

You can find full details of our natural protocol of treating odema problems in our book:

How to Rid Swelling without Medications which will be printed in the United States soon.

We can draw the main guidelines of our protocol as follows:

1. Juice that Heal: Noni, Tomato, **Cranberry**, Aloe Vera and Celery juice can be helpful.

2. Food that Heal: Lettuce, Cucumber, Cabbage and Tomato are also helpful. Pomegranate, Ginger, Almonds and Walnuts and **Grape Seed Extract, Baking Powder are well known by their effects on improving** odema.

3. Herbs that Heal: Eating 1 tsp of flax seed and black seed every morning for 3 months is good for odema. The Indian herb; Shilajit is one of the best herbs for odema. **Dandelion and Tribulus terrestris are also very useful.**

4. Milk that Heals: Camel milk (as narrated by Prophet Mohammad (PBUH) offers endless health benefits. One of those is treating odema problems. My patients who took 2 glasses of camel milk daily or our food supplement **Reno Tech** for 3 months found miracle results for both odema and sex!!!!!

5. Herbal Tea that Heals: Hundreds of odema cases who took our herbal tea; Lymph **Tea** which is simply composed of Celery, Linden and **Coriander seed** for 3-6 weeks could easily solve odema problem without medications!!!!!

6. Food Supplemnts that Heal: Many patients obtained excellent results by using our food supplement named: **Reno Tech** which contains a number of **diuretic** herbs including **Coriander seed!!!!**Together with **chlorophyll** supplement.

CORIANDER AND PIMPLES, BLACKHEADS AND DRY SKIN

Pimples and blackheads can occur for a variety of reasons, such as bacteria, hormonal fluctuations and excess oil. While there are a variety of different medications available to treat all kinds of acne, you don't have to use such products to clear your skin. With a regular skin care regime and some simple home remedies, you can get rid of pimples and blackheads quickly, without using acne-treatment products.

A teaspoon for coriander juice, mixed with a pinch of turmeric powder, is an effective remedy for pimples, blackheads and dry skin.

Natural Methods of Treating Pimples, Blackheads and Dry Skin:

You can find full details of our natural protocol of treating acne problems in our book: **How to Rid Pimples, Blackheads and Dry Skin without Medications** which will be printed in the United States soon.

We can draw the main guidelines of our protocol as follows:

1. Juice that Heal: Coriander juice (mixed with turmeric powder or mint juice) is used as a treatment for Pimples, Blackheads and Dry Skin: applied to the face in the manner of toner.

2. Food that Heal: Lettuce, Cucumber, Curcumin are also helpful. Apple Cider Vinegar, **Baking Powder is well known by their effects on improving** Pimples, Blackheads and Dry Skin.

3. Herbs that Heal. Coriander, Aloe Vera: Neem, Turmeric, Papaya., Calendula, Propolis is one of the best herbs for Pimples, Blackheads and Dry Skin.

4. Milk that Heals: Camel milk (as narrated by Prophet Mohammad (PBUH) offers endless health benefits. One of those is treating Pimples, Blackheads and Dry Skin. My patients who took 2 glasses of camel milk daily for 3 weeks found miracle results for Pimples, Blackheads and Dry Skin!!!!!

5. Herbal Tea that Heals: Many Pimples, Blackheads and Dry Skin cases who took our herbal tea composed of Lemon Balm and Coriander seed for 3 weeks could easily solve their Pimples, Blackheads and Dry Skin without medications!

6. Food Supplemnts that Heal:, Vitamin B3, Zinc, MSM together with chlorophyll food supplement.

7. Essential Oils that Heal: Citronelol, a component of essential oils in **coriander**, is an excellent antiseptic. In addition, other components have anti microbial and healing effects which have beautiful effects on Pimples, Blackheads and Dry Skin. Our oil: **Relax U:** was successfully used by Pimples, Blackheads and Dry Skin patients!!!

8. Soap that Heals: Dr.Mansour Miracle Nano Soap was successfully used by hundreds who got rid of their Pimples, Blackheads and Dry Skin in 7-10 days!!!!

9. Ceam that Heals: Many Pimples, Blackheads and Dry Skin patients used our Cellu Tech and 14 in One got rid of their Pimples, Blackheads and Dry Skin in 3 weeks.

10.Bath that Heals: Many patients cured their Pimples, Blackheads and Dry Skin by using a 15-minute baking powder bath together with our dead sea salt or mud!!!

CORIANDER AND PROSTATE HEALTH

The prostate is the male sex gland is the size of a chestnut in the shape of a doughnut through which the urinary tract runs. The prostate is also in charge of discharging sperm during ejaculation semen is mainly made of prostatic fluid. The symptoms of renal failure include <u>edema</u>, which is an accumulation of fluid characterized by swelling, and a decrease in urination. Other symptoms may include a general ill feeling, exhaustion and headaches. Often, a person with renal failure does not experience any symptoms.

Benign prostatic hypertrophy is the gradual enlargement of the prostate it's very a common problem for men more than 50 years of age and 75% of men more than seventy years of age suffer from it. Is cause by hormonal changes in the body as we age, later in life men's production of dihydrotestosterone increases leading to an over production of prostate cells, this makes the prostate grow.

From the phytochemical composition of coriander we can notice a number of chemical compounds forming Coriander act as excellent **diuretic** anti-inflammatory agents, which clearly means that coriander is a good candidate to be safely used for prostate health.

Coriander serves both as an herb and a spice. It is a healing herb that is used effectively in different parts of the globe. While Indians use it for its anti-inflammatory properties, many other nations use this perennial herb for prostate health.

Plant sterols and sterolins – plant sterols are fatty compounds, abundant in seeds, nuts and legumes. It is believed that sterols are active ingredients in saw palmetto and pygeum africanum, which attribute these herbs with their BPH relieving properties. The most abundant plant sterol **beta-sitosterol** has been currently used in Europe for BPH treatment. In one report, beta-sitosterol was found to induce prostate cancer cell apoptosis (death) in humans. Pytosterols have shown to significantly improve BPH's urological symptoms and urine flow in four double-blind, placebo-controlled studies. Laboratory and animal studies have shown that when plant sterols and sterolins are administrated together, they enhance the immune system and help improve hormonal balance

Many prostate cases used **Coriander seed tea** from kitchen together with our powerful **Prosta Tech** food supplement and after 3-6 months they got excellent results without any medications!!!!!

Triphala – a combination of three fruit extracts: terminalia chebula, terminalia belerica and emblica officinalis. This combination has been used traditionally to improve digestion, elimination and overall body toning. Triphala contains anti-inflammatory, antioxidant and anti-cancerous compounds including tannins, bioflavonoids and vitamin C and is very useful for prostate health.

Natural Methods of Treating Heart Problems:

You can find full details of our natural protocol of treating prostate enlargement in our book:

How to Fix Your Prostate without Medications which will be printed in the United States soon.

We can draw the main guidelines of our protocol as follows:

1. Juice that Heal: Noni, Tomato, Cranberry, Aloe Vera and Celery juice can be helpful.

2. Food that Heal: Asparagus Soup, Lettuce, Nopal Cactus and Tomato lycopene are also helpful. Garlic is useful to improve the prostate health by the scientific research. Bee Pollens shown remarkable success improving 80% of the cases and curing 40% of them within 6 months, **Pomegranate, Baking Powder are well known by their effects on improving prostate health.Pumpkis Seed plays an important role.**

3. Herbs that Heal: Eating 1 tsp of flax seed and black seed every morning for 3 months is good for Prostate. The Indian herb; Shilajit is one of the best herbs for prostate. Corn Silk, Uva Ursi, Myrrh, Milk Thistle, Neem, Dandelion, Goldenseal, **Saw Palmetto** and **Tribulus terrestris,** Guggul, **Nettle Root,** Sandalwood **are also very useful.**

4. Milk that Heals: Camel milk (as narrated by Prophet Mohammad (PBUH) offers endless health benefits. One of those is treating prostate problems. My patients who took 2 glasses of camel milk daily or our food supplement **Prosta Tech** for 3-6 months found miracle results for both prostate and sex!!!!!

5. Herbal Tea that Heals: Hundreds of kidney cases who took our herbal tea; Pros Tea which is simply composed of Corn Silk, Crataeva nurvala and **Coriander** seed for 3-6 months could easily improve prostate health without medications!!!!!

6. Food Supplemnts that Heal: Many patients obtained excellent results by using our food supplement named: **Prosta Tech** which contains a number of **diuretic** herbs including **Coriander** seed!!!!Together with **chlorophyll** supplement.

CORIANDER AND PROSTATITIS

The prostate is the male sex gland is the size of a chestnut in the shape of a doughnut through which the urinary tract runs. The prostate is also in charge of discharging sperm during ejaculation semen is mainly made of prostatic fluid.

Prostatitis is an inflammation in the prostate gland; this is a very common problem for men of all ages. Bacteria from different parts of the body infect the prostate and that causes prostatitis. Once infected the prostate swells restricting the flow of urine and causing urine retention. There are three types of prostatitis: acute infectious prostatitis, chronic infectious prostatitis, and noninfectious prostatitis

From the phytochemical composition of coriander we can notice a number of chemical compounds forming Coriander act as excellent **diuretic** anti-inflammatory agents, which clearly means that coriander is a good candidate to be safely used for prostatitis.

Coriander serves both as an herb and a spice. It is a healing herb that is used effectively in different parts of the globe. While Indians use it for its anti-inflammatory properties, many other nations use this perennial herb for prostatitis

Many prostatitis cases used **Coriander** seed tea from kitchen together with our powerful **Prosta Tech2** food supplement and after 3-6 months they got excellent results without any medications!!!!!

Natural Methods of Treating Heart Problems:

You can find full details of our natural protocol of treating prostatitis in our book:

How to Fix Prostatitis without Medications which will be printed in the United States soon.

We can draw the main guidelines of our protocol as follows:

1. Juice that Heal: Radish, Pomegranate, Tomato, Cranberry, Aloe Vera and Celery juice can be helpful.

2. Food that Heal: Asparagus Soup, Nopal Cactus, Cabbage and Tomato lycopene are also helpful. Garlic is useful to improve the prostatitis by the scientific research.

3. Herbs that Heal: Eating 1 tsp of flax seed and black seed every morning for 3 months is good for Prostatitis. The Indian herb ; Shilajit is one of the best herbs for prostatitis.Corn Silk, Uva Ursi, Myrrh, Milk Thistle, Neem, Dandelion, Goldenseal, **Saw Palmetto** and **Tribulus terrestris,** Guggul, **Nettle Root,** Sandalwood **are also very useful.**

4. Milk that Heals: Camel milk (as narrated by Prophet Mohammad (PBUH) offers endless health benefits. One of those is treating prostate problems. My patients who took 2 glasses of camel milk daily or our food supplement **Prosta Tech2** for 3-6 months found miracle results for both prostatitis and sex!!!!!

5. Herbal Tea that Heals: Hundreds of prostatitis cases who took our herbal tea ;Pros Tea which is simply composed of Corn Silk, Crataeva nurvala and **Coriander** seed for 3-6 months could easily improve heart functions without medications!!!!!

6. Food Supplemnts that Heal: Many patients obtained excellent results by using our food supplement named: **Prosta**

Tech2 which contains a number of **diuretic** herbs including **Coriander** seed, Amla berries'

7. Vitamins that Heal: Vitamin B17, Vitamin C, Zinc and Vitamin E

8. Magnet that Heals: While most of chemical and herbal formulas failed to cure prostatitis my patients were successful in curing their prostatitis by using the Russian Magnetic Prostate Rod after 13 years of continuous usage of antibiotics. For details please refer to our book: **How to Fix Your Prostatitis without Medications**

CORIANDER AND PSORIASIS

Major Causes of Psoriasis

Psoriasis is considered a non-curable, long-term (chronic) skin condition. It has a variable course, periodically improving and worsening. Sometimes psoriasis may clear for years and stay in remission. Some people have worsening of their symptoms in the colder winter months. Many people report improvement in warmer months, climates, or with increased sunlight exposure especially the balanced UV layer found in the Dead Sea area in Jordan and Palestine.

Following is a list of causes or underlying that could possibly cause Psoriasis includes: Genetic predisposition, Factors that may aggravate psoriasis include stress, excessive alcohol consumption, and smoking, Withdrawal of systemic steroids, Drugs, including salicylates, iodine, lithium, phenylbutazone, oxyphenbutazone, trazodone, penicillin, hydroxychloroquine, calcipotriol, interferon-alpha, and interferon-beta injection Strong, irritating topical, including tar, anthralin, steroids under occlusion, and zinc pyrithione in shampoo, Infections, Sunlight or phototherapy, Cholestatic jaundice, Calcium deficiency, Sudden withdrawal of oral corticosteroids (prednisone).

It has been found that psoriasis patients suffer from folic acid and Vitamin B12 deficiency.

Coal tar is probably the oldest psoriasis remedy known to medicine and its origins as an anti- psoriasis treatment but it is famous to cause skin cancer!!!

Some famous products in the market use Salicylic acid inside creams but it causes many side effects and skin irritation!!!!

Coriander serves both as an herb and a spice. It is a healing herb that is used effectively in different parts of the globe. While Indians use it for its anti-inflammatory properties, many other nations use this perennial herb for psoriasis.

Natural Methods of Treating Psoriasis:

You can find full details of our natural protocol of treating psoriasis problems in our book:

How to Rid Psoriasis in 4 Weeks without Medications which will be printed in the United States soon.

We can draw the main guidelines of our protocol as follows:

1. Juice that Heal: Coriander juice (mixed with turmeric powder or mint juice) is used as a treatment for psoriasis as a drink, and applied to the psoriasis areas.

2. Food that Heal: Lettuce, Cucumber, Curcumin are also helpful. Apple Cider Vinegar, **Baking Powder is well known by their effects on improving** psoriasis.

3. Herbs that Heal. Coriander, Aloe Vera: Neem, Turmeric, Papaya., Calendula, Propolis is one of the best herbs for psoriasis.

4. Milk that Heals: Camel milk (as narrated by Prophet Mohammad (PBUH) offers endless health benefits. One of those is treating psoriasis. My patients who took 2 glasses of camel milk daily for 4 weeks found miracle results for psoriasis!!!!!

5. Herbal Tea that Heals: Hundreds of psoriasis cases who took our herbal tea composed of Turmeric and Coriander seed for 4 weeks together with our cream; Psoria Tech did easily solve their psoriasis without medications!!And one of the difficult cases was a female medical doctor who suffered for several years of her severe Rheumatic Psoriasis and finally got rid of both Rheumatoid and Psoriasis!!!

6. Food Supplemnts that Heal:, Vitamin B3, <u>Zinc</u>, MSM together with chlorophyll food supplement.

7. Essential Oils that Heal: Citronelol, a component of essential oils in **coriander**, is an excellent antiseptic. In addition, other components have anti microbial and healing effects which do not let psoriasis go worse.

8. Soap that Heals: Dr.Mansour Miracle Nano Soap was successfully used by hundreds who got rid of their psoriasis in 4 weeks!!!!

9. Ceam that Heals: Many psoriasis patients used our Psoria Tech Cream which is very essential to rid of psoriasis in 4-6 weeks.

10. Bath that Heals: Many patients cured their psoriasis by using a 15-minute baking powder bath together with our Dead Sea mud!!!

CORIANDER AND SEX

From the phytochemical composition of coriander we can notice a number of chemical compounds forming Coriander act as a diuretic and as a vasodilator agents, which clearly means that coriander is a good candidate to be safely used for sex.

Who would think that you could help cure a low sex drive with coriander? Of course you should always consult your physician if you have any ongoing sexual dysfunction, but **coriander can be a quick fix**. It's <u>natural</u> and healthy with no side effects typically associated with Erectile Dysfunction prescription medication.

Coriander is one of the oldest herbs and spices on record. Coriander was mentioned in the Bible comparing it to Manna. Coriander seeds have been found in ruins dating back to 5000 B.C... As an <u>aphrodisiac</u> coriander is famous from its mention in the "Arabian Nights" where it was used in a concoction to cure a merchant of impotence!!!!

The Chinese believed coriander would offer provide immortality and used it in many love spells to help cure sexual impotence. The Greeks and Romans also prescribed to coriander in their love potions and it's even mentioned in Sanskrit.

The Middle Ages, there was a drink that was created by Hippocrates that became a staple at many wedding parties. It contains several herbs such as **coriander**, cardamom, clove, ginger, and cinnamon. This **drink is called "Hippocras"**. This drink was eventually banned because it stimulated the libido too much. Now you can create and drink this drink yourself to help cure a low <u>sex drive</u>.

Natural Methods of Treating Hypertension:

You can find full details of our natural protocol of treating sex impotence in our book:

How to be a Real Man without Medications which will be printed in the United States soon.

We can draw the main guidelines of our protocol as follows:

1. Juice that Heal: Acai, Strawberry, Tomato, and Celery juice can be helpful.

2. Food that Heal: Banana and Potato (rich in potassium), Cocoa, Dark Chocolate, Yogurt and Apple are also helpful... Honey and Cinnamon are useful for low sex drive by the scientific research.

3. Herbs that Heal: Eating 1 tsp of khella and flax seed every morning for 3 months is said to prevent hypertension due to heredity factors. They also cure hypertension due to obesity, as both seeds have weight reducing properties.

4. Milk that Heals: Camel milk (as narrated by Prophet Mohammad (PBUH) offers endless health benefits. One of those is treating impotence and infertility. Camel milk is said to be the Viagra of the Future". My patients who took 2 glasses of camel milk daily or our food supplement: **Camel Tech** for 3 months found miracle results for sex!!!!!

5. Herbal Tea that Heals: Hundreds of low libido cases who took our herbal tea ;**Heart & Love Tea** which is simply composed of Hibiscus, Cinnamon, Mint and **Coriander seed**

for 3-6 months could easily restore their sexual power to normal without medications!!!!!

6. Food Supplemnts that Heal: Many patients obtained excellent results by using our food supplemenst named: **ViaTech** and Vita-X which contain a number of stimulating herbs including **Coriander seed!!!!**

Hippocras Sex Drink

- 3/4 Gallon Grape juice
- 1 Cup Honey
- 2 Tablespoons cinnamon
- 2 Tablespoons Fresh Grated Ginger
- 1 Tablespoon Nutmeg
- 1 Tablespoon Mace
- 1 Tablespoon Cloves
- 1 Tablespoon Cardamom
- 1 Tablespoon Coriander
- 1 Tablespoon Cayenne

Mix all spices together and set aside. Heat the grape juice to just below boiling. Add spices to the juice and allow cooling. Pour the mix into air tight glass containers and set it in a cool dark place for one week. Strain the juice and return to air tight containers. Let this concoction rest for about one month before drinking. It will keep unopened for years, about four days after opening.

CORIANDER AND SMALLPOX

From World Health Organization (WHO): Smallpox is an acute contagious disease caused by variola virus.

Smallpox, which is believed to have originated over 3, 000 years ago in India or Egypt, is one of the most devastating diseases known to humanity. For centuries, repeated epidemics swept across continents, decimating populations and changing the course of history. In some ancient cultures, smallpox was such a major killer of infants that custom forbade the naming of a newborn until the infant had caught the disease and proved it would survive.

Smallpox killed Queen Mary II of England, Emperor Joseph I of Austria, King Luis I of Spain, Tsar Peter II of Russia, Queen Ulrika Elenora of Sweden, and King Louis XV of France.

The disease, for which no effective treatment was ever developed, killed as many as 30% of those infected. Between 65–80% of survivors were marked with deep pitted scars (pockmarks), most prominent on the face. Blindness was another complication. In 18th century Europe, a third of all reported cases of blindness were due to smallpox.

One teaspoon fresh **coriander juice**, mixed with 1 or 2 seeds of banana, given once daily regularly, for a week is a very effective preventive measure against small pox. It is believed that putting fresh leaf juice in the eyes, during an attack of small pox, prevents eye damage.

Eating Coriander promotes a faster curing process when suffering from smallpox while reducing the pain simultaneously.

Egyptians used Henna to treat smallpox.

Turmeric was successfully used to rid of smallpox and chickenpox.

The Herbs that are famous to treat smallpox are: Garlic, Bistort, Black Cohosh, Goldenseal, Hyssop, Lobelia, Tansy And Yarrow.

Our cream; All in One is very useful for smallpox well as gangrene ad fungus.

Our oil mix of Lavender and Coriander are very useful too.

CORIANDER AND SORE THROAT

Sore throats are one of the most common reasons why people see a doctor. In the United States, sore throats account for more than 18 million visits to the doctor each year.

One of the easiest, least expensive home remedies to treat a sore throat is the following herbal formula:

1 ½ cups of water

1 table spoon of Coriander seed

Directions:

1-Soak coriander inside water over night.

2-Discard coriander seed next morning.

3-Gargle with water and let it reach inside your throat

4-Throw water away. You will feel much better in less than 1 hour.

5-Repeat the same process many times till you are OK.

Other home remedies:

Gargle with salty water many times till symptoms disappear.

Use Zinc.

Use Bee Propolis which is equivalent to 132 antibiotics.

Uses our oil mix RELAX U externally.

Slippery Elm, Licorice, Hyssop, Elecampane, Ginger, Marshmallow, Honey Water, and Sage.

CORIANDER AND TRIGLYCERIDES

Triglycerides are the chemical form in which most fat exists in food as well as in the body. They're also present in blood plasma and, in association with cholesterol, form the plasma lipids.

Triglycerides in plasma are derived from fats eaten in foods or made in the body from other energy sources like carbohydrates. Calories ingested in a meal and not used immediately by tissues are converted to triglycerides and transported to fat cells to be stored. Hormones regulate the release of triglycerides from fat tissue so they meet the body's needs for energy between meals.

Everyone with high triglycerides needs to keep it under control, but it may be even more important for some groups of people, such as

- People with a family history of early heart disease
- People with high blood pressure
- People with diabetes
- People with obesity
- People with continuous stress
- Males over age 45
- Females over age 55
- Smokers

From the phytochemical composition of coriander we can notice a number of chemical compounds forming Coriander act as anti-lipid and anti- triglycerides agents, which clearly means that coriander is a good candidate to be safely used for high triglycerides.

Coriander serves both as an herb and a spice. It is a healing herb that is used effectively in different parts of the globe. While Indians use it for its anti-inflammatory properties, many other nations use this perennial herb for high cholesterol and triglycerides.

Coriander was given to rats that had been fed a high-fat and high- triglycerides <u>diet</u>. The spice lowered total <u>cholesterol</u> and triglycerides significantly!!!!

CardiovascularDiseaseandBloodLipids

Coriander lowers cholesterol and triglyceride levels, helping to reduce the risk of atherosclerosis and thereby heart attack and stroke. It does this through two mechanisms: by inhibiting the uptake of these lipids in the intestines, and by enhancing their breakdown and excretion.

In for high triglyceride management it has been shown that <u>Coriander acts as an anti-lipid agent and also helps in the vasodilatation of veins!!</u>

Many high cholesterol cases used **Coriander seed tea** from kitchen together with my powerful **Choles Tech** food supplement and after 3 months they got excellent results without any medications!!!!!

Natural Methods of Treating High Triglyceride:

You can find full details of our natural protocol of treating high triglyceride in our book:

How to Lower Your High Triglyceride to Normal without Medications which will be printed in the United States soon.

We can draw the main guidelines of our protocol as follows:

1. Juice that Heal: Acai, Tomato, Cucumber, and Celery juice can be helpful.

2. Food that Heal: Dark Chocolate, Peanut Butter, Lettuce, Cucumber, Sunflower seeds, Yogurt and Tomato are also helpful. **Garlic** is useful to lower the blood high triglyceride by the scientific research. **Apple cider vinegar** to lower triglyceride: It is said that an 8oz.apple juice with a tablespoon of apple cider vinegar will lower cholesterol and triglyceride. Almonds and **Walnuts** are very famous for lowering triglyceride. **Grape Seed Extract is well known by its effect in lowering** triglyceride. **Royal Jelly** is a beautiful food to lower triglyceride.

3. Herbs that Heal: Eating 1 tsp of flax seed and black seed every morning for 3 months is said to prevent high triglyceride due to heredity factors. They also cure high triglyceride due to obesity, as both seeds have weight reducing properties. The Indian famous herb; Guggul.

4. Milk that Heals: Camel milk (as narrated by Prophet Mohammad (PBUH) offers endless health benefits. One of those is treating high triglyceride. Camel milk is said to be the vasodilator of the Future". My patients who took 2 glasses of camel milk daily or our food supplement: **CholesTech** for 3 months found miracle results for both high triglyceride and sex!!!!!

5. Herbal Tea that Heals: Hundreds of high triglyceride cases who took our herbal tea ;**Heart & Love Tea** which is simply composed of Cinnamon, Fenugreek and **Coriander seed** for 3-6 months could easily reduce their high cholesterol to normal without medications!!!!!

6. Food Supplements that Heal: Many patients obtained excellent results by using our food supplement named: **Choles Tech** which contains a number of anti-lipid herbs including **Coriander seed!!!!**

7.Exercise that Heals: One of the most important factors that helped thousands of people to reduce high triglyceride is to perform daily exercise together with **Royal Jelly** and **L-LYSINE** amino acid from health stores.

In a research paper authored by V. Chithra and S. Leelamma entitled "Hypolipidemic effect of coriander seeds" The effect of the administration of coriander seeds (Coriandrum sativum) on the metabolism of lipids was studied in rats fed a high fat diet with added cholesterol. The spice had a significant hypolipidemic action. The levels of **total cholesterol and triglycerides decreased significantly i**n the tissues of the animals of the experimental group which received coriander seeds.

A recent experiment from the Biochemistry Department at the University of Kerala, in India, studied the effects of coriander seeds on rats that had been fed a very high-fat, high-cholesterol diet. Researchers saw significant drops in total cholesterol and triglyceride levels in the rats as lipid was broken down faster and eliminated.

CORIANDER AND ULCER

Peptic ulcer disease refers to painful sores or ulcers in the lining of the stomach or first part of the small intestine, called the duodenum.

What Causes Ulcers?

No single cause has been found for ulcers. However, it is now clear that an ulcer is the end result of an imbalance between digestive fluids in the stomach and duodenum. Ulcers can be caused by:

• Infection with a type of bacteria called Helicobacter pylori **(H. pylori)** which also causes **stomach cancer!!!**

• Use of painkillers called no steroidal anti-inflammatory drugs (NSAIDs), such as aspirin, naproxen (Aleve, Anaprox, Naprosyn, and others), ibuprofen (Motrin, Advil, Midol, and others), and many others available by prescription. Even aspirin coated with a special substance can still cause ulcers.

• Excess acid production from gastrinomas, tumors of the acid producing cells of the stomach that increases acid output.

Coriander helps cure ulcer, inflammation and spasm.

As for drinks, one should avoid alcoholic drinks completely.

Coriander serves both as an herb and a spice. It is a healing herb that is used effectively in different parts of the globe. While Indians use it for its anti-inflammatory properties, many other nations use this perennial herb for peptic ulcer.

As for drinks, one should avoid alcoholic drinks completely during mouth ulcer attack.

Coriander serves both as an herb and a spice. It is a healing herb that is used effectively in different parts of the globe. While Indians use it for its anti-inflammatory properties, many other nations use this perennial herb for peptic ulcer Natural Methods of Treating Ulcer:

You can find full details of our natural protocol of treating peptic ulcer problems in our book:

How to Fix Ulcer without Medications which will be printed in the United States soon.

We can draw the main guidelines of our protocol as follows:

1. Juice that Heal: Licorice, Cabbage juice represents a miracle cure for ulcer.

2. Food that Heal: Cherry, Lettuce, Cucumber, Cabbage are also helpful. Pomegranate, Ginger, Almonds, Walnuts, **Baking Powder are well known by their effects on improving** peptic ulcer.

3. Herbs that Heal: Eating 1 tsp of Fenugreek, Aloe Vera, Ginger, Lemon Balm, Chamomile, Peppermint, Licorice and black seed every morning for 3 weeks is good for mouth ulcer. The Indian herb; Shilajit is one of the best herbs for peptic ulcer.

4. Milk that Heals: Camel milk (as narrated by Prophet Mohammad (PBUH) offers endless health benefits. One of those is treating peptic ulcer. My patients who took 2 glasses of camel milk daily for 3 months found miracle results for both peptic ulcer and sex!!!!!

5. Herbal Tea that Heals: Hundreds of mouth ulcer cases who took our herbal tea ;**Diges Tech Tea** which is simply composed of Licorice, Alfalfa, Pomegranate Peels, Propolis and **Coriander seed** for 3 weeks could easily solve their peptic ulcer without medications!!!!!

6. Food Supplemnts that Heal: Many patients obtained excellent results by using our food supplement named: **Stomach Care** which contains a number of herbs including **Coriander seed!!!!** Together with **chlorophyll** supplement.

7. Essential Oils that Heal: Citronelol, a component of essential oils in **coriander**, is an excellent antiseptic. In addition, other components have anti microbial and healing effects which do not let wounds and ulcers in the mouth go worse. They aid healing up of ulcers and freshen up the breath

CORIANDER AND URINARY TRACT INFECTION (UTI)

Urinary Tract Infection (UTI) is an infection by the bacteria of the urinary tract which includes kidney, ureters, bladder or urethra. This bacterium enters the opening of the urethra and procreates in the urinary tract causing urinary tract infection. This can be very painful and a major cause of distress in your life. If it is not contained in the earlier stages it is likely to spread to your kidneys, which can become a serious health issue. The infection of the bladder can develop into cystitis- a very common problem faced by women. Urinary Tract Infection can infect anyone but women are more susceptible to this disease. Children too suffer from this disorder but the headcount is very low in comparison to adults. Sexual intercourse is another reason for urinary tract infection.

From the phytochemical composition of coriander we can notice a number of chemical compounds forming coriander act as excellent diuretic anti-inflammatory agents, which clearly means that coriander is a good candidate to be safely used for Urinary Tract Infection!!!.

Coriander serves both as an herb and a spice. It is a healing herb that is used effectively in different parts of the globe. While Indians use it for its anti-inflammatory properties, and hence for UTI.

Many stories about using coriander seed tea as a diuretic **and** anti-inflammatory tool for **UTI!!!!** Many Qatari and Saudi UTI patients; got rid of it within 4 weeks only!!!! After starting taking coriander tea together with our food supplement **URI TECH and Cranberry Juice** without any medications!!!!!

Natural Methods of Treating UTI Problems:

You can find full details of our natural protocol of treating UTI problems in our book:

How to Rid UTI in 3 Weeks without Medications which will be printed in the United States soon.

We can draw the main guidelines of our protocol as follows:

1. Juice that Heal: Cranberry and drinking 2-3 glasses water on empty stomach can be very helpful.

2. Food that Heal: Lettuce, Cucumber, Cabbage are also helpful. Pomegranate**, Baking Powder is well known by their effects on improving** UTI.

3. Herbs that Heal: Eating 1 tsp of corn silk and cinnamon with honey every morning for 3 weeks is good for UTI the Indian herb; Shilajit is one of the best herbs for UTI. Dandelion and Tribulus **terrestris are also useful.**

4. Milk that Heals: Camel milk (as narrated by Prophet Mohammad (PBUH) offers endless health benefits. One of those is treating UTI problems. My patients who took 2 glasses of camel milk daily or our food supplement **Uri Tech** for 3 months found miracle results for both UTI and sex!!!!!

5. Herbal Tea that Heals: Hundreds of gout cases who took our herbal tea; Uri **Tech Tea** which is simply composed of Corn Silk, Parsley and Coriander seed for 3-6 weeks could easily solve their UTI problem without medications!!!!!

6. Food Supplemnts that Heal: Many patients obtained excellent results by using our food supplement named: **Uri Tech** which contains a number of diuretic herbs including **Coriander seed!!!!** Together with chlorophyll **supplement.**

7. Essential Oils that Heal: You can make an essential oil by using equal parts of Coriander, sandalwood, frankincense and juniper. Mix all these ingredients to make an oil to be rubbed over your bladder area. Continue this massaging technique for three to four days once the symptoms subside

8. Avoid irritant foods: A diet which consists of processed food like cheese, chocolate, dairy products should be avoided. You should also avoid spicy food, caffeine, alcohol and cigarettes which otherwise is also harmful. Avoid carbonated drinks like beer, soda or any other drink with fizz, and Aspartame which is one of the artificial sweeteners.

CORIANDER AND WEIGHT LOSS

Being overweight is a common condition, especially where food supplies are plentiful and lifestyles are sedentary. As much as 64% of the United States adult population is considered either overweight or obese, and this percentage has increased over the last four decades.

Excess weight has reached epidemic proportions globally, with more than 1 billion adults being either overweight or obese-Increases have been observed across all age groups.

Causes

Factors which may contribute to this imbalance include:

- Limited physical exercise
- Overeating
- Poor nutrition
- Genetic predisposition
- Hormonal imbalances (e.g. hypothyroidism)
- Metabolic disorders, Eating disorders (such as binge eating)
- Alcoholism
- Stress
- Insufficient or poor-quality sleep
- Psychotropic medication
- Smoking cessation

In some cases, insulin dependent diabetes can cause weight gain in some sufferers, as opposed to type II diabetes which mostly comes on as a result of being overweight.

From the phytochemical composition of coriander we can notice a number of chemical compounds forming Coriander act as excellent **diuretic** agents, which clearly means that coriander is a good candidate to be safely used for weight loss!!!.

Coriander serves both as an herb and a spice. It is a healing herb that is used effectively in different parts of the globe. While Indians use it for its anti-inflammatory properties, many other nations use this perennial herb for kidney health.

Many obesity cases used **Coriander seed tea** from kitchen together with our powerful **SlimTech** food supplement and after 3 months they got excellent results without any medications!!!!!

Natural Methods of Treating Heart Problems:

You can find full details of our natural protocol of treating heart problems in our book:

How to be Slim without Medications which will be printed in the United States soon.

We can draw the main guidelines of our protocol as follows:

1. Juice that Heal: Tomato**, Cranberry**, Cabbage and Celery juice can be helpful.

2. Food that Heal: Asparagus Soup, Lettuce, Cucumber, Cabbage and Tomato are also helpful. **Yogurt, Ginger, Almonds** and **Sunflower** and **Grape Seed Extract, Baking Powder are well known by their effects on losing weight.**

3. Herbs that Heal: Eating 1 tsp of flax seed and cinnamon every morning for 3 months is good for obesity. The Indian herb; **Shilajit** is one of the best herbs for obesity. **Dandelion,**

<u>Anise, Senna,</u> <u>Caralluma Fimbriata and Licorice</u> are also very useful.

4. Milk that Heals: Camel milk (as narrated by Prophet Mohammad (PBUH) offers endless health benefits. One of those is treating obesity problems. My patients who took 2 glasses of camel milk daily or our food supplement **Reno Tech** for 3 months found miracle results for both obesity and sex!!!!!

5. Herbal Tea that Heals: Hundreds of obesity cases who took our herbal tea ;**Slimming Tea** which is simply composed of Anise, Fennel, Senna and **Coriander seed** for 3-6 months could easily reduce weight without medications!!!!!

6. Food Supplemnts that Heal: Many patients obtained excellent results by using our food supplement named: **Slim Tech** which contains a number of **diuretic** herbs including **Coriander seed!!!!** Together with **kelp** supplement.

CORIANDER AS AN EFFICIENT HEAVY METALS DETOX SORBENT

Removal and preconcentration of inorganic and methyl mercury from aqueous media using a sorbent prepared from the plant Coriandrum sativum **CORIANDER.**

A sorbent prepared from the plant Coriandrum sativum, commonly known as **coriander or Chinese parsley**, was observed to remove inorganic ($Hg2+$) and methyl mercury ($CH3Hg+$) from aqueous solutions with good efficiency. Batch experiments were carried out to determine the pH dependency in the range 1–10 and the time profiles of sorption for both the species. Removal of both the forms of mercury from spiked ground water samples was found to be efficient and not influenced by other ions. Column experiments with silica-immobilized coriander demonstrated that the sorbent is capable of removing considerable amounts of both forms of mercury from water. The sorption behavior indicates the major role of carboxylic acid groups in **binding the mercury**. The studies suggest that the sorbent can be used for the decontamination of inorganic and methyl mercury from contaminated waters.

Delicious recipe for heavy-metal cleansing:

CORIANDER CHELATION PESTO

4 cloves garlic

1/3 cup Brazil nuts (selenium)
1/3 cup sunflower seeds (cysteine)
1/3 cup pumpkin seeds (zinc, magnesium)
2 cups packed fresh coriander (cilantro, Chinese parsley) (vitamin A)
2/3 cup flaxseed oil
4 tablespoons lemon juice (vitamin C)
2 tsp dulse powder
Sea salt to taste

Process the coriander and flaxseed oil in a blender until the coriander is chopped. Add the garlic, nuts and seeds, dulse and lemon juice and mix until the mixture is finely blended into a paste. Add a pinch to sea salt to taste and blend again. Store in dark glass jars if possible. It freezes well, so purchase coriander in season and fill enough jars to last through the year.

Coriander has been proven to **chelate toxic metals from our bodies** in a relatively short period of time. Combined with the benefits of the other ingredients, this recipe is a powerful tissue cleanser. Two teaspoons of this pesto daily for three weeks is purportedly enough to increase the **urinary excretion of mercury, lead and aluminum,** thus effectively removing these toxic metals from our bodies. We can consider doing this cleanses for three weeks at least once a year. The pesto is delicious on toast, baked potatoes, and pasta.

CORIANDER CABBAGE MIRACLE SLIMMING SOUP

Ingredients:

450g onions
1/2 Savoy cabbage (about 400g)
2 tablespoons olive oil
2 red or 4 green chillies, finely chopped
4 garlic cloves, finely chopped
About 5 cm fresh root ginger, peeled and chopped
2 tablespoons **coriander** seeds, crushed
800ml good vegetable stock
400ml tin of coconut milk
Bunch of fresh **coriander**, chopped
Juice of 3 limes
Salt and black pepper.

Finely chop the onions and very finely shred the cabbage, either by hand or by using the finest slicing disc on a food processor.
Heat the oil in a pan, add the onion and cabbage, and cook them over a moderate heat for a couple of minutes before adding the chillies, garlic, ginger and coriander seeds. Continue cooking for about 5 minutes, stirring regularly, until the onion and cabbage are tender but still have a bite to them.

Bring the stock to the boil in a separate pan and add to the vegetables. Simmer for 5 minutes, then add the coconut milk, half of the fresh coriander, the lime juice and finally salt and pepper.

Serve the soup with extra coriander to taste.

This soup is famous for its slimming miracle results.

CORIANDER, LICE AND DANDRUFF

Head **lice** are tiny insects that live on the scalp. They can be spread by close contact with other people. These **lice** only live in hair and occasionally eyebrows and eyelashes.

Dandruff is a form of dermatitis caused by fungal infection of the skin and hair follicles. Dandruff is also known as Seborrheic Dermatitis, Cradle Cap, Seborrhea and Seborrheic eczema. Dandruff is characterized by scaly skin which is shed in the form of flakes. Dandruff if not treated can lead to loss of hair and eye infections. Guava fruit extract is very effective in the treatment of dandruff. Regular application of Guava fruit extract helps to cure dandruff. Guava fruit extracts are a natural alternative to commonly used as anti-fungus.

Coriander oil is one of the best remedies to kill lice on head.

Coriander oil is one of the best solutions for dandruff problems and it is included

In our **Magic Hair Oil** and **Smart Shampoo**.

Other Effective Home Remedies for dandruff:

Henna pasted with water and applied on scalp.

Coconut, Pineapple and Lime: Grated coconut and pineapple and mixed thoroughly with lime (squeeze it) and coconut water. Then sieved and used to wash the hair every five days.

5 to 10 Guava fruits crushed into a fine paste. And applied twice daily for a week. The Dandruff is resolved in a week.

Neem oil is used after shampoo on daily basis. It is good for both lice and dandruff.

Spinach infused in water over night and then used twice daily till dandruff is cured.

Lime juice is rinsed on hair twice daily.

Apple Cider Vinegar is mixed with any shampoo to cure dandruff.

Olive Oil is very helpful to treat dandruff.

Olive Oil mixed with Almond oil is fast in curing dandruff.

Tea Tree Oil is also helpful to treat dandruff.

Aloe Vera Gel is used for 10 minutes on scalp and then washed by shampoo.

For head lice problem wash your hair with vinegar. It will kill all the nits in two days. Apply coconut oil to your head after shampoo and condition. Add ten to fifteen drops of tea tree oil into shampoo bottle and use it daily. Rub Listerine mouth wash on your head. This will kill all the lice. Massage your head with mayonnaise and comb it after 2 hours. This will kill all the lice and their eggs. Apply a mixture of lemon and butter on your head, wait for 15 seconds and then rinse your head.

Camphor oil and Lemon oil are excellent for lice treatment.

Our OIL mix: Lice Tech Oil is very fast in killing lice in minutes.

CORIANDER, NAUSEA AND VOMITING

Nausea and vomiting are not diseases, but rather are symptoms of many different conditions, such as infection ("stomach flu"), food poisoning, motion sickness, overeating, blocked intestine, illness, concussion or brain injury, appendicitis, and migraines. Nausea and vomiting can sometimes be symptoms of more serious diseases such as heart attacks, kidney or liver disorders, central nervous system disorders, brain tumors, and some forms of cancer.

Coriander cures nausea and tendency to vomit: Boiled coriander water with <u>sugar</u> candy is beneficial. 33 ml of the juice of green coriander leaves checks vomiting. **Vomiting during pregnancy can also be treated**. It should be taken frequently.

Home remedies for nausea and vomiting:

Effective home remedy for vomiting using Cauliflower: It contains substances which are alkaline. It purifies blood. Eating cooked or raw cauliflower is **beneficial in bloody vomiting.** The patients of TB should definitely take it.

Natural home remedy for vomiting using Mint leaves: Take half a cup of the juice of mint leaves at an interval of every two hours. You can add lemon juice to it. Frequent use of the chutney of green coriander leaves and mint leaves is quite **beneficial for vomiting**.

Herbal home remedy for vomiting using Neem: Grind 25 gms. Of neem leaves, mix with water, strain and drink. It can **check all types of vomiting**.

Simple home remedy for vomiting: Vomiting during pregnancy-soak 50 gms. Rice in 250 ml. water. After half an hour put 5 gms. Coriander seeds in it. Then after ten minutes stir and strain. Divide it into four parts and take them as four doses in one day. It will provide relief **to the pregnant woman from vomiting**.

Good home remedy for vomiting: Grind two cloves and give it with honey to the pregnant woman, in case of vomiting. Sucking a roasted clove **treats vomiting**. Whenever vomiting takes place, suck a roasted clove.

Effective home remedy for vomiting: Soak ripe tamarind in water, then mash, strain and drink it. It will **check vomiting.**

Natural home remedy for vomiting: Soak gram in water at night. Take the water next morning. This wills **cures vomiting in pregnancy**, the woman should be given sattu made of roasted gram

Diet tips for vomiting

Banana: Eating ripe bananas checks bloody vomiting.

Pistachio: Eating four pistachios will vomiting and nausea.

Harad: Taking harad powder mixed with honey controls vomiting.

Honey: Taking onion juice mixed with honey checks vomiting.

Water-melon: In case of heart burn after meals and yellowish vomit, take water-melon juice with sugar candy in the morning.

Onion: Taking 2 tsp. of the mixed juice of ginger and onion can control vomiting.

Sugarcane: In case of bilious vomiting, taking sugarcane juice mixed with honey will be beneficial.

Cinnamon: Take cinnamon powder mixed with honey to get relief from bilious vomiting.

Basil: The juice of basil leaves checks vomiting. Taking honey mixed with the juice of basil leaves provides relief from vomiting and nausea.

CORIANDER PERFUMES AND COLOGNES

Coriander oil is obtained by steam distillation of ripe fruits of Coriandrum Sativum. It is mainly cultivated in Eastern Europe.

Coriander is an essential composition in many perfumes and cologne famous names; for example:

Paco Rabanne Perfume - Xs Elle Eau De Toilette Spray-100ml/3.3oz for Women

Opium 6.6 oz body lotion:

This lotion contains coriander, clove, bay leaf and is accented with vetiver

Soir De Lune by Sisley Eau De Parfum:

It has top notes of mandarin, lemon, and peach, bergamot, **coriander**, nutmeg, and pepper.

Fragrance personality: Warm, sweet, comforting. This long-lasting fragrance is filled with the exotic indulgence of creamy coconut on a tropical island.

Family: fruity

Base notes: coconut, vanilla, milky sandalwood

Fragrance Notes: Top: Coconut, **Coriander** and Coconut Milk. Heart: Coconut. Base: Coconut, Vanilla, and Milky Sandalwood.

Coriander Perfume for Women:

Coriander EDT SP 1.1 Oz. Jean Couturier Designer Perfume. Coriander perfume for women.

Bergamot Coriander Solid Perfume:by ZAJA Natural – 1 By ZAJA Natural Solid Perfumes.

Demeter Fragrance Library cologne splash coriander: Little is known about the origins of the coriander plant, although it is generally thought to be native to the Mediterranean and parts of southwestern Europe. Experts believe its use dates back to at least 5, 000 BC.

Coriander & Coca Cola Secret Formula

The Coca-Cola formula is The Coca-Cola Company's secret recipe for Coca-Cola. As a publicity marketing strategy started by Robert W. Woodruff, the company presents the formula as one of the most closely held trade secrets in modern business that only a few employees know or have access to. Experienced perfumers and food scientists - today aided by modern analytical methods - can easily identify the composition of food products, a fact that is further supported by the many cola flavorings and competing soft drinks like Pepsi.

Coca-Cola formula - Recipe 1. This recipe is attributed to a sheet of paper found in an old formulary book owned by Coca-Cola inventor, John S. Pemberton, just before his death (U.S. measures): 1 oz caffeine citrate 3 oz citric acid 1 fl oz extract vanilla 1 qt lime juice 2½ oz flavoring (**coriander**) 30 lb (14 kg) sugar 4 fl oz fluid extract of coca (decocainized flavor essence of the coca leaf) 2½ gal water Caramel sufficient.

Excessive Body Heat Home Remedy Using Water and Coriander

An extremely hot weather sometimes results in overheated body temperatures in people predisposed to it. This can result in improper digestion, restlessness, and a general feeling of unwellness.

Directions for Use: Soak about 10gms of coriander seeds overnight in water that has been pre-boiled and cooled. Drink this as first thing in the morning for 2 weeks.

(From: mamaherb.com)

Grapefruit and Coriander Bath Oil

100ml almond oil
20ml wheat germ oil
30 drops grapefruit essential oil
30 drops coriander essential oil
Mix above together in a glass bottle before mixing two tablespoons into a warm bath.
This bath is famous for stress and insomnia!!
It is used for 30 minutes 3 times weekly and it is called RELAX U BATH.

Phytochemical Compounds Inside Coriander & Their Effects on Health

Chemical Compounds and their Activities in Coriander

Here is a list of the most important chemical compounds found in coriander together with their benefit effects on different health issues (from Duke's Phytochemical Database):

Antiparkinsonian
Antipneumonic
Antiretinotic
Antirheumatic
Antiseptic
Antishingles
Antispasmodic
Antistress
Antitumor (Gastric)
Antitumor (Lung)
Antiulcer
Antiviral
Asthma-preventive
Beta-Adrenergic
Receptor Blocker
Cancer-Preventive
Cardioprotective
Cold-preventive
Detoxicant
Diuretic
Hypocholesterolemic
Hypotensive
Immunomodulator
Immunostimulant
Vasodilator

AntiCrohn's
Antidepressant
Antidiabetic
Antidote (Cadmium
Antidote (Lead)
Antieczemic
Antiedemic
Antifatigue
Antigallstone
Antigastritic
Antigingivitic
Antihepatitic
Antihepatotoxic
Antiherpetic
Antihistaminic
Antihypertensive
Antiinfertility
Antiinflammatory
Antimenopausal
Antimigraine
Antiobesity
Antiorchitic
Antiosteoarthritic
Antiosteoporotic
Antioxidant

ALPHA-PINENE
Antibacterial
Antiflu
Antiinflammatory
Antipneumonic;
Antiseptic
Antispasmodic;
Antiviral
Cancer-Preventive

ASCORBIC-ACID
Aldose-Reductase-
Inhibitor
Analgesic
Angiotensin-Receptor-
Blocker
AntiAGE
Antiallergic
Antialzheimeran
Antiarthritic
Antiasthmatic
Antiatherosclerotic
Antibacterial
Anticataract
Anticold

Cancer-Preventive
Cardioprotective
Diuretic
Hypocholesterolemic
Hypotensive
Laxative
Vasodilator

LIMONENE
AChE-Inhibitor
Antiasthmatic
Antibacterial
Anticancer
Antiflu
Antiinflammatory
Antilymphomic
Antimetastatic
(Stomach)
Antiobesity
Antiseptic
Antispasmodic
Antitumor;Antitumor
(Breast)
Antitumor (Colon)
Antitumor (Pancreas)
Antitumor (Prostate)
Antitumor (Stomach)
Antiviral
Cancer-Preventive
Chemopreventive
Cholesterolytic
Detoxicant
Expectorant
FLavor
Immunomodulator

LINALOL

Antihypertensive
Antimenopausal
Antiobesity
Antiosteoporotic
AntiPMS
Antirheumatic
Antistress
Diuretic
Hypocholesterolemic
Hypotensive
Laxative
Vasodilator

CHROMIUM
AntiAGE
Antiatherosclerotic
Antidiabetic
Antidote (Lead)
Antifatigue
Antiobesity
Antitriglyceride
Cardioprotective
Energizer
Hypocholesterolemic
Hypoglycemic
Hypotensive
Immunomodulator
Insulinogenic
Memorigenic

FIBER
Angiotensin-Receptor-
Blocker
Antidiabetic
Antihypertensive
Antiobesity
Antitumor
Antiulcer
Beta-Blocker

**BETA-
SITOSTEROL**
Angiogenic
Antibacterial
Anticancer (Breast)
Anticancer (Cervix)
Anticancer (Lung)
Antiedemic
Antiestrogenic
Antifertility
Antihyperlipoproteinae
mic
Antiinflammatory
Antileukemic
Antilymphomic
Antioxidant
Antiprostatadenomic
Antiprostatitic
Antitumor (Breast)
Antitumor (Cervix)
Antitumor (Lung)
Antiviral
Cancer-Preventive
Hepatoprotective
Hypocholesterolemic
Hypoglycemic
Hypolipidemic
Pesticide
Spermicide

CALCIUM
Antiallergic
Antianxiety
Antiarrhythmic
Antiarthritic
Antiatherosclerotic
Antidepressant
Antidote (Lead)

Antioxidant
Flavor
Hypercholesterolemic
Pesticide

PENTOSANS
Anti-prostatitis
Anti-bladder
inflammation
Anti-interstitial cystitis

PETROSELINIC-ACID
Anti-inflammatory
Anti-colic
Anti-cholesterol
Anti-lipid

POTASSIUM
Antiarrhythmic
Antidepressant
Antifatigue
Antihypertensive
Antispasmodic
Antistroke
Beta-Blocker
Cardioprotective
Diuretic
Hypotensive
Vasodilator

Antidiabetic
Antidysmenorrheic
Antiepileptic
Antifatigue
Antifibromyalgic
Antigastrotic
Antihypertensive
Antiinflammatory
Antiinsomniac
Antimenopausal
AntiMS
Antiretinopathic
Antispasmodic
Antistress
Antistroke
Cardioprotective
Diuretic
Hypocholesterolemic
Hypotensive
Immunomodulator
Insulinogenic
Laxative
Vasodilator

OLEIC-ACID
Antiinflammatory
Cancer-Preventive
Dermatitigenic
Hypocholesterolemic
Perfumery

PALMITIC-ACID
Antifibrinolytic

Anti-diabetic,
Hypoglycemic, Anti-lipid

LINOLEIC-ACID
5-Alpha-Reductase-Inhibitor
Antiacne
Antialopecic
Antiarteriosclerotic
Antiarthritic
Anticoronary
Antieczemic
Antihistaminic
Antiinflammatory
AntiMS
Antiprostatitic
Cancer-Preventive
Hepatoprotective
Hypocholesterolemic
Immunomodulator

MAGNESIUM
Antiaggregant
Antialcoholic
Antianginal
Antianxiety
Antiarrhythmic
Antiarthritic
Antiasthmatic
Antiatherosclerotic
Anticoronary
Antidepressant

We can summarize the phytonutrients of coriander by the following list:

It contains:

Vitamin A, C, E (Alpha Tocopherol) and K

Thiamine
Zinc

Potassium	Vitamin B6
Copper	Riboflavin
Manganese	carotene
Selenium	Niacin
proteins	Folate
fat	Pantothenic Acid
fiber	minerals like Calcium
carbohydrates	Iron
water	Magnesium
	Phosphorus

It is very clear from the list of chemical compounds present in coriander and their action that coriander inner composition offers us huge number of health benefits for:

Diabetes, Cholesterol, Triglycerides, Gout, Kidney, Liver, Heart, Ulcer, Gallbladder, Prostate, Joints, Cancer, High Blood Pressure, Weight Loss, Asthma......etc.

The chapters of the book show us in details about these health benefits.